Squamous Cell Cancer of the Neck

T0331112

Contemporary Issues in Cancer Imaging

A Multidisciplinary Approach

Series Editor

Rodney H. Reznek
Cancer Imaging, St Bartholomew's Hospital, London

Editorial Adviser

Janet E. Husband
Diagnostic Radiology, Royal Marsden Hospital, Surrey

Current titles in the series

Cancer of the Ovary
Lung Cancer
Colorectal Cancer
Carcinoma of the Kidney
Carcinoma of the Esophagus
Carcinoma of the Bladder

Forthcoming titles in the series

Prostate Cancer
Pancreatic Cancer
Interventional Radiological Treatment of Liver Tumors
Gastric Cancer
Primary Carcinomas of the Liver
Breast Cancer

Squamous Cell Cancer of the Neck

Edited by
Robert Hermans

Series Editor
Rodney H. Reznek

Editorial Adviser
Janet E. Husband

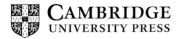
CAMBRIDGE
UNIVERSITY PRESS

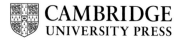

Shaftesbury Road, Cambridge CB2 8EA, United Kingdom

One Liberty Plaza, 20th Floor, New York, NY 10006, USA

477 Williamstown Road, Port Melbourne, VIC 3207, Australia

314–321, 3rd Floor, Plot 3, Splendor Forum, Jasola District Centre, New Delhi – 110025, India

103 Penang Road, #05–06/07, Visioncrest Commercial, Singapore 238467

Cambridge University Press is part of Cambridge University Press & Assessment,
a department of the University of Cambridge.

We share the University's mission to contribute to society through the pursuit of
education, learning and research at the highest international levels of excellence.

www.cambridge.org
Information on this title: www.cambridge.org/9780521886918

First published 2008

A catalogue record for this publication is available from the British Library

ISBN   978-0-521-88691-8   Hardback

Contents

The color plates are between pages 34 and 35.

Contributors

Dominique Chevalier
Service d'O.R.L et de chirurgie
cervico-faciale
Hôpital Claude Huriez
Lille, France

Vincent F. Chong
Department of Diagnostic Radiology
National University of Singapore
Singapore

Pierre R. Delaere
Department of Otorhinolaryngology,
Head and Neck Surgery
University Hospitals Leuven
Leuven, Belgium

Frédérique Dubrulle
Service de Radiologie
Hôpital Claude Huriez
Lille, France

Lawrence E. Ginsberg
Department of Diagnostic Radiology
M. D. Anderson Cancer Center
University of Texas
Houston, Texas
USA

Robert Hermans
Department of Radiology
University Hospitals Leuven
Leuven, Belgium

Ann D. King
Department of Diagnostic Radiology and Organ
Imaging
Faculty of Medicine
The Chinese University of Hong Kong
Shatin, Hong Kong
China

Sandra Nuyts
Department of Radiation Oncology
University Hospitals Leuven
Leuven, Belgium

Philippe Puech
Service de Radiologie
Hôpital Claude Huriez
Lille, France

Vincent Vander Poorten
Department of Otorhinolaryngology,
Head and Neck Surgery
University Hospitals Leuven
Leuven, Belgium

Raphaëlle Souillard
Service de Radiologie
Hôpital Claude Huriez
Lille, France

Series Foreword

Imaging has become pivotal in all aspects of the management of patients with cancer. At the same time, it is acknowledged that optimal patient care is best achieved by a multidisciplinary team approach. The explosion of technological developments in imaging over the past years has meant that all members of the multidisciplinary team should understand the potential applications, limitations and advantages of all the evolving and exciting imaging techniques. Equally, to understand the significance of the imaging findings and to contribute actively to management decisions and to the development of new clinical applications for imaging, it is critical that the radiologist should have sufficient background knowledge of different tumors. Thus, the radiologist should understand the pathology, the clinical background, the therapeutic options and the prognostic indicators of malignancy.

Contemporary Issues in Cancer Imaging – A Multidisciplinary Approach aims to meet the growing requirement for radiologists to have detailed knowledge of the individual tumors in which they are involved in making management decisions. A series of single subject issues, each of which will be dedicated to a single tumor site, edited by recognized expert guest editors, will include contributions from basic scientists, pathologists, surgeons, oncologists, radiologists and others.

While the series is written predominantly for the radiologist, it is hoped that individual issues will contain sufficient varied information so as to be of interest to all medical disciplines and to other health professionals managing patients with cancer. As with imaging, advances have occurred in all these disciplines related to cancer management and it is our fervent hope that this series, bringing together expertise from such a range of related specialties, will not only promote the understanding and rational application of modern imaging but will also help to achieve the ultimate goal of improving outcomes of patients with cancer.

Rodney H. Reznek

Preface to Squamous Cell Cancer of the Neck

Squamous cell cancer is one of the most common neoplasms in the head and neck. In this complex anatomical environment, accurate staging of neoplasm is a challenging task. As these lesions originate from the mucosal lining, the clinician is often able to detect their presence; however, it may be difficult or impossible to appreciate, based on the physical examination, the entire submucosal tumor extension, or the possible regional and distant disease spread.

Modern imaging tools provide a reliable visualization of the head and neck tissues. Carefully performed cross-sectional imaging allows an accurate evaluation of the local and regional cancer extent, and the exclusion or detection of distant metastasis.

The radiologist is an important member of the multidisciplinary team managing patients with head and neck cancer. Recent evolutions, such as positron emission tomography–computed tomography (PET–CT) and diffusion-weighted magnetic resonance imaging, have further increased the impact of imaging in oncological patient care. The added value of existing imaging techniques, such as CT, in choosing the optimal treatment strategy and in monitoring tumor response, is now scientifically established.

The purpose of this book is to review state-of-the-art imaging in head and neck squamous cell cancer, and to describe its role within the overall diagnostic and therapeutic management of this disease.

Robert Hermans

1

Introduction: epidemiology, pathology and clinical presentation

Vincent Vander Poorten

In general in the head and neck, two major groups of malignant neoplasms can be recognized. A smaller but important group of neoplasms can be described as "glandular neoplasms," the majority arising in the thyroid, a minority in the salivary glands. These tumors are not considered in this chapter. This chapter deals specifically with the largest group of malignancies, so-called squamous cell carcinoma (SCC) of the head and neck (HNSCC). These account for about 90% of all head and neck cancers [1] and originate in the mucosal membranes of the upper aerodigestive tract. Squamous cell carcinoma also arises from the skin. Skin cancer is generally considered a separate entity, as is skin cancer of the head and neck.

Head and neck neoplasia observed less frequently include localized lymphoma, soft tissue and bone sarcomas, and neuroectodermal tissue tumors (paraganglioma, olfactory neuroblastoma, neuroendocrine carcinoma, malignant melanoma). As this volume deals specifically with HNSCC, the reader is referred to specific oncological literature for information on other neoplasms.

This chapter deals with the epidemiology, pathology and clinical presentation of premalignant and malignant head and neck neoplasms.

Epidemiology: frequency measures and risk factors

Incidence

Head and neck cancer, excluding skin cancer and Hodgkin and non-Hodgkin lymphoma, is the sixth most frequent cancer in the world. Approximately 500 000 new malignancies of the mucous membranes are registered per year (oral and pharyngeal cancer: 363 000 new cases and 200 000 deaths yearly; laryngeal cancer: 136 000 new cases and 73 500 deaths yearly) [2]. This represents 6% of the global incidence of

Squamous Cell Cancer of the Neck, ed. Robert Hermans. Published by Cambridge University Press.
© R. Hermans 2009.

Table 1.1. Proportion of malignant tumors (% of total) arising in the major anatomic sites in the Flemish population of Belgium

Type	Male (%)	Female (%)
Oral SCC	33	34
Oropharyngeal SCC	11	7
Hypopharyngeal SCC	7	3
Laryngeal SCC	34	10
Nasopharyngeal–paranasal sinuses	6	5
Salivary gland	4	7
Thyroid	5	34

SCC, squamous cell carcinoma.

cancer. In the European Union in 1997, 5% of the global cancer burden encountered was caused by oral, pharyngeal and laryngeal cancer [3]. The larynx and oral cavity are most frequently involved, as indicated by the population-based numbers of the Flemish Cancer Registry in Belgium (Table 1.1) [4]. Overall, the incidence is dependent on gender and geography. In HNSCC, there is a definite male preponderance. For example, a male/female ratio of 10/1 is observed in the incidence of laryngeal SCC [5]. There is an important geographical variation in the incidence of specific head and neck subsites for cancer. For example, hypopharyngeal SCC is typically more frequent in northern France (10/100 000 males per year) than in the USA (2/100 000 males per year). The yearly incidence of laryngeal cancer in northern Spain (20/100 000) is approximately 200 times the incidence in certain regions in China (0.1/100 000) [6]. Apart from differences in genetic susceptibility, a different prevalence of strong risk factors (e.g., tobacco use, Calvados drinking) largely explains these geographical differences. Also a large part of the observed differences in incidence among races (lower incidence in Caucasian versus African Americans [7]), and observed gender differences, can be attributed to marked differences in exposure to risk factors [8].

Risk factors

Chronic use of tobacco and alcohol is the main cause of the development of HNSCC. Epidemiologically, the strong association with the induction of the disease and the very high prevalence of the factors among the population explain the strength and the impact of the causal relationship that is observed. Tobacco and

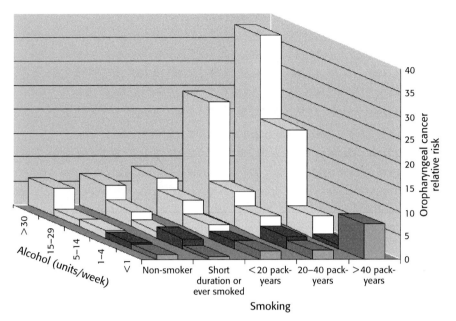

Axis labels (from figure):

Oropharyngeal cancer relative risk (right axis): 0, 5, 10, 15, 20, 25, 30, 35, 40

Alcohol (units/week): >30, 15–29, 5–14, 1–4, <

Smoking: Non-smoker, Short duration or ever smoked, <20 pack-years, 20–40 pack-years, >40 pack-years

Fig. 1.1. Relative risk for development of oral and pharyngeal cancer for males according to amount of tobacco and alcohol used. (Based on data from W. J. Blot *et al. Cancer Res* 48 (1988), 3282–3287, with permission.)

alcohol are independent risk factors that act in a multiplicative way when used together. Figure 1.1 illustrates the 5.8 times increased risk for development of oral and pharyngeal cancer in non-smokers who consume 30 or more drinks per week and the 7.4 times increase in risk observed in non-drinking smokers with a history of smoking 20 cigarettes per day for 40 years. A person combining these two bad habits multiplies these relative risks to a 38 times increased risk [9]. After stopping the use of tobacco, the risk for oral mucosal dysplasia and cancer takes 15 years to reach the level of the population that never smoked [10].

Tobacco contains the carcinogens aldehydes, polycyclic aromatic hydrocarbons and nitrosamines. Nitrosamines are alkylating agents that induce mutational events. Alcohol acts as a solvent, enhancing permeation of toxic substances in tobacco into the cells of the mucosa. Alcohol is directly carcinogenic following mucosal enzymatic reduction (by alcohol dehydrogenase) to acetaldehyde. The oro- and hypopharyngeal mucosal surfaces especially are at risk for alcohol-induced carcinogenesis [11]. The mucosa of the glottic larynx does not have direct contact with the carcinogen and, therefore, only very high alcohol consumption is found to increase HNSCC risk independently. Alcohol intake creates exposure to other carcinogenic compounds such as tannin in wine and nitrosodimethylamine in beer. Furthermore, high intake of these beverages implies nutritional deficiencies, which also increase the risk of HNSCC development by losing the proven protective effect of high intake of fruits and vegetables. A diet rich in fresh fruit and vegetables has been estimated to reduce the incidence of HNSCC by 50–70% [12]. Especially protective are dark yellow vegetables, citrus fruits and carotene-rich vegetables (fresh tomatoes, pumpkins, carrots). These vegetables contain crucial antioxidant micronutrients such as vitamin C, vitamin E, beta-carotene, and flavonoids [13]. High-fibre intake [12] and olive oil [14] are also suggested to have protective effects.

All the factors enumerated so far are associated with socio-economic status, which, therefore, itself is also strongly associated with the development of HNSCC. Three out four patients with HNSCC are located in the lower social classes, in terms of level of education and income. One in three patients has no partner and one in six patients is unemployed at the time of diagnosis. This social situation is strongly linked to the combination of the direct risk factors tobacco, alcohol, poor dietary habits and lower level of oral hygiene. Once HNSCC has developed, people in lower socio-economic groups will find their way to the health system with more difficulty because of less education, and will present with more advanced stages of disease. Stage at presentation is the strongest negative prognostic factor for outcome of treatment in HNSCC. Treatment of advanced disease often has a serious physical and psychological impact. A serious effort is needed to adapt to the resulting altered body image, to integrate back into society and to realise the change in lifestyle needed to reduce the risk of a second primary HNSCC. Unfortunately, following treatment, patients in lower social classes have less support to face this challenge. Rehabilitation is often very difficult for many of these patients [15]. A lower socio-economic environment is a strong negative prognostic factor for the results of treatment and also for survival in general because of the lasting effect of the comorbidities that result from the former lifestyle (e.g., liver disease, pulmonary insufficiency, atherosclerosis).

Viral infections also have been implicated in the pathogenesis of HNSCC [14]. Human papilloma virus (HPV) DNA is prevalent in approximately 50% of patients with oral cancer and in 72% of those with oropharyngeal cancer. Relative risks up to 6.2 for development of oral cancer have been reported, and recently a relative risk of 12 for the development of oropharyngeal cancer has been confirmed. Type 16 HPV seems particularly associated with the development of oropharyngeal SCC, both in patients with and patients without the risk factors tobacco and alcohol [16]. It does not seem unrealistic to expect an effect of HPV vaccination on the future incidence of these tumors. Epstein–Barr virus (EBV) has been strongly associated with nasopharyngeal cancer. Antibody titers for EBV are much higher in cases than in controls, and biopsy specimens of undifferentiated nasopharyngeal carcinoma are 100% EBV positive and monoclonal for this virus [17]. Following treatment,EBV antibody titers are used to follow patients for disease recurrence. Patients infected with the human immunodeficiency virus (HIV) have an increased risk of developing HNSCC and Kaposi sarcoma.

Occupational factors have been implicated in HNSCC development. Working in industry with higher exposure to aromatic amines and phenoxy herbicides creates an elevated risk for all sites. The rate of development of SCC of the sinonasal tract is increased 250 times in workers exposed to nickel [18]. Among environmental factors, chronic sun exposure causes development of skin and lip cancer.

Pathology

The first step is to identify the tumor as SCC. The pathologist then has to identify prognostic factors such as the grade of differentiation, perineural or vascular invasion, and the assessment of the resection margins following surgery.

Epithelial neoplasms of the mucous membranes

Premalignant lesions

Premalignant lesions will usually not be visualized on routine imaging studies. Different forms of leukoplakia are distinguished: homogeneous leukoplakia and non-homogeneous leukoplakia (Figs. 1.2 and 1.3, respectively).

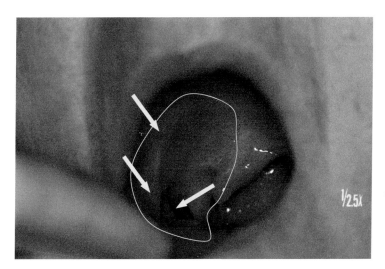

Fig. 1.2. Erythroplakia (encircled) with areas of nodular leukoplakia (arrows) of the tonsil, glossotonsillar sulcus, anterior tonsillar pillar and hard and soft palates. Color version in plate section.

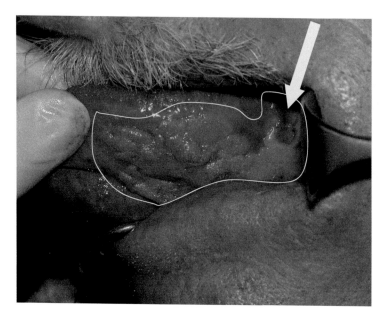

Fig. 1.3. Non-homogeneous leukoplakia (encircled) with area of invasive carcinoma (arrow) of the lateral tongue. Color version in plate section.

Leukoplakia is "a white plaque or patch that cannot be characterized, clinically or histopathologically, as any other disease" [19]. It should be impossible to scrape off the lesion, unlike candidal patches. Another condition for this diagnosis is that the lesion should not be associated with any physical (frictional keratosis, candidal leukoplakia) or chemical agent, except tobacco.

Homogeneous leukoplakia is the most frequent observation, corresponding microscopically to hyperortho- or hyperparakeratosis, and rarely shows associated dysplasia. The yearly rate of malignant transformation of homogeneous leukoplakia is estimated to be between 2% and 6% in the Western world and is higher in older, female patients and when the lesion persists for a longer time.

Non-homogeneous leukoplakia (nodular leukoplakia, erythroplakia, proliferative verrucous leukoplakia) is less frequently observed but is usually associated with dysplasia and is, therefore, much more prone to becoming invasive [20]. The rate of malignant transformation in non-homogeneous (speckled) leukoplakia (Fig. 1.3) and erythroplakia can exceed 50% [21].

Microscopically, epithelial hyperplasia, dysplasia and carcinoma in situ are sought. Dysplasia is described as "mild" where there is an increased number of mitotic figures and an abnormal cytological appearance only in the basal layer of the epithelium, whereas suprabasal mitosis and cytological abnormality indicates "moderate" dysplasia. In "severe" dysplasia, the atypical cells with mitotic activity

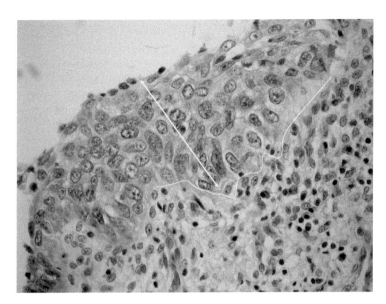

Fig. 1.4. Carcinoma in situ. Loss of an orderly nuclear mosaic pattern, increased nuclear/cytoplasmic ratio and an irregular random nuclear placement can be observed in all suprabasal cells (double arrow). Yellow line shows lamina basalis of epithelium. Color version in plate section. (Courtesy of Raf Sciot.)

and abnormal cytological features such as loss of an orderly nuclear mosaic pattern, decreased nuclear/cytoplasmic ratio and an irregular random nuclear placement, can be observed from the basal to the most superficial layers. The term carcinoma in situ indicates that all suprabasal cells are abnormal but signs of invasion can still not be detected (Fig. 1.4).

Malignant lesions

Entities seen less frequently but with a specific clinical behavior are verrucous carcinoma, papillary SCC, basaloid SCC and sarcomatous SCC, increasingly aggressive in that order. Verrucous carcinoma is an exophytic papillomatous SCC that is low grade, very well differentiated and without known potential for regional or distant metastasis [22]. Papillary SCC displays an exophytic growth with a poorly differentiated cell layer lining a central fibrovascular core. The behavior of this type of tumor is more aggressive than verrucous carcinoma in that metastases occur. Basaloid SCC and sarcomatoid SCC are highly aggressive variants of SCC.

Most of the malignancies of the mucous membranes are simply called "invasive squamous cell carcinoma" and can be graded as well, moderately and poorly differentiated, paralleling the amount of keratin formation by cells (Fig. 1.5). Cells in SCC, by definition, produce intercellular bridges. Absence of these intercellular bridges is one of the features of undifferentiated carcinoma of the upper aerodigestive tract. This type of tumor occurs most frequently in the nasopharynx.

Table 1.2. Histopathological negative prognostic factors in HNSCC head and neck squamous cell carcinoma

---

Increasing (p)TNM classification: size of primary tumor, number/laterality of positive nodes, size of largest node

Vascular invasion

Perineural growth

Involved resection margins, e.g., less than 5 mm is considered "close margins" in oral cancer

Increasing tumor thickness

Invasive front, i.e., infiltration of the submucosa (Fig. 1.5)

Loss of differentiation

Endophytic worse than exophytic growth pattern

Field cancerization

Increasing mitotic index

Presence of extracapsular spread in metastatic lymph nodes

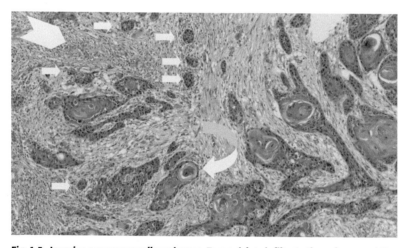

Fig. 1.5. Invasive squamous cell carcinoma. Tumor islets infiltrate the submucosal tissue (small arrows); there is an intense mononuclear inflammatory reaction (large arrowhead) and the formation of keratin pearls (curved arrow). Color version in plate section. (Courtesy of Raf Sciot.)

The most important microscopic findings to be determined following resection of a primary HNSCC and the regional lymph nodes are listed in Table 1.2. These findings are negatively associated with prognosis, so their routine determination during microscopical analysis contributes to the decision making concerning the need for further therapy, the particular postoperative radiotherapy and whether this is with or without chemotherapy.

Clinical presentation

The clinical presentation of a patient with this specific group of malignancies typically depends on the anatomical site of origin of the tumor. Usually, there will be involvement of the local sensory innervation or function of the aerodigestive tract, resulting in typical symptoms.

Each site of origin also has a regional lymphatic drainage system and, therefore, depending on the site of origin, regional metastatic disease in the neck is common at the time of presentation [23]. Conversely, in patients where the only symptom is a mass in the neck, the site of regional metastasis can point to the primary site. The typical association between a specific site of origin and the corresponding preferred level of regional lymph node metastasis is shown in Fig. 1.6. The locoregional extent is typically summarized in the UICC TNM classification, the last edition dating from 2002 [24]. The classification rules for attributing a HNSCC lesion to a specific T category differ according to the anatomic subsite in which the neoplasm arises, and this will be discussed in the dedicated subsequent chapters. The N classification is universal for all sites except for nasopharyngeal carcinoma, as will also be discussed later.

Clinical presentation at diagnosis

Patients with *glottic* laryngeal cancer tend to present at an earlier stage, given the effect of even a small vocal cord lesion on voice quality. This early presentation in combination with a relatively sparse lymphatic drainage corresponds to a low incidence of regional metastasis at presentation. This accounts for the observed good prognosis of HNSCC at this site. Five-year survival rates following radio-therapy or surgery range from 70 to 100% (Fig. 1.7) [25].

As pointed out under "risk factors", many patients with *supraglottic laryngeal, oral* and *pharyngeal* cancer will present at an advanced stage of their disease because of the late occurrence of symptoms. A comparison of this marked difference in stage at presentation of patients with glottic versus supraglottic cancer in the Memorial Sloan-Kettering Cancer Center [26] is shown in Fig. 1.8. Supraglottic laryngeal cancer will produce hoarseness only late in its development, by mucosal extension to the vocal cord, the arytenoid or the cricoarytenoid joint, or by submucosal extension to the paraglottic space. Other typical symptoms of advanced glottic and supraglottic laryngeal cancer, but also of oro- and hypopharyngeal cancer, are respiratory obstruction, hemoptysis and referred otalgia. Dysphagia and odynophagia

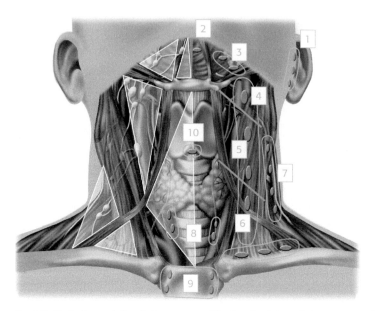

Fig. 1.6. Typical association between a specific site of origin and the corresponding likely level of regional lymph node metastasis in cancer of the head and neck. 1. Parotid nodes: primary tumors in forehead and anterior scalp skin, in the parotid gland. 2. Level Ia, medially from anterior belly digastric: primary in lower lip, lower alveolar crest, anterior floor of mouth. 3. Level Ib between anterior and posterior belly digastric: primary in skin of face and nose, oral cavity, paranasal sinuses, submandibular gland. 4. Level II, inferior of posterior belly digastric, above hyoid bone, medial of sternocleidomastoid muscle (above upper green line): primary in nasopharynx, oral cavity, oropharynx, supraglottic larynx, hypopharynx. 5. Level III, below hyoid, above caudal border cricoid, medial of sternocleidomastoid muscle: primary in nasopharynx, larynx, hypopharynx, cervical esophagus, thyroid gland (below upper green line and above lower green line). 6. Level IV, below cricoid, above clavicle, medial of sternocleidomastoid muscle: primary in nasopharynx, thyroid, esophagus, lung, breast. 7. Level V, laterally from sternocleidomastoid muscle: primary in nasopharynx, thyroid, esophagus, stomach, lung, breast. 8. Level VI, central compartment above thoracic inlet, lymph nodes: primary in larynx, hypopharynx, cervical esophagus or thyroid. 9. Level VII, upper mediastinal nodes above innominate artery: primary in thyroid or subglottic larynx, hypopharynx, cervical esophagus. 10. Prelaryngeal, delphian node: primary in larynx or in thyroid. Color version in plate section. (Courtesy of Pierre Delaere.)

are typically observed in supraglottic laryngeal, oro- and hypopharyngeal cancer, but all usually relatively late in the development of the disease. As already discussed, once symptoms occur, the often compromised social situation will make access to the medical system more difficult and further delay diagnosis and advance the stage at diagnosis.

Patients with *oral cavity* SCC will usually present with an exophytic (Fig. 1.9) or endophytic (Fig. 1.10) ulcerative lesion; endophytic tumors are associated with

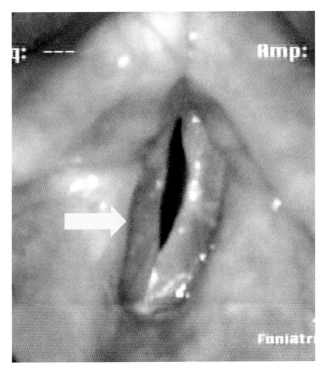

Fig. 1.7. Vocal cord carcinoma causes hoarseness relatively early in the course of disease, resulting in a relatively high proportion of early stage disease at presentation. Hoarseness results from impaired mucosal wave and vibratory capacity of the vocal cord (right affected here, arrowed) compared with the normal mucosal wave which will occur on the opposite side. Color version in plate section.

more extensive submucous spread than initially would be expected. Typical symptoms at presentation are pain, reduced tongue movement interfering with speech or oral transport of food, impaired denture fitting or reduced mouth opening (trismus) following infiltration of the masticatory muscles. For oral cavity SCC with advanced T classification (T3–T4), 50–75% of patients will have neck disease at presentation [27].

Oropharyngeal cancer likewise is associated with a high proportion (66%) of patients with neck disease at presentation [27]. Local pain in the throat or referred otalgia (Fig. 1.11), feeling of a lump in the throat and impaired mobility of the tongue and palate are other presenting symptoms, but usually only after the tumor volume is quite extensive. In the same way, the advanced stage at presentation of patients with *nasosinusal* and *nasopharyngeal* carcinomas is because symptoms only occur when a significant local tumor volume has formed or significant surrounding structures have become invaded. For nasosinusal cancer, typical "early" symptoms of tumor spread still confined to the nasal cavity are (unilateral) nasal obstruction (Fig. 1.12), epistaxis or sinusitis. These symptoms remain present in more advanced stage of disease, of course, but then become associated with

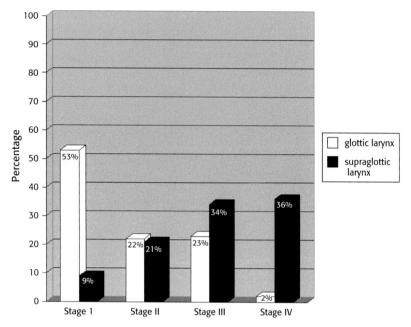

Fig. 1.8. Stage distribution of laryngeal cancer at presentation according to site of origin (black, glottic larynx; white, supraglottic larynx). Patients presenting at the Head and Neck Service of Memorial Sloan-Kettering Cancer Center New York, J. Shah and S. G. Patel 1985–2000. (Modified with permission from *Head and Neck Surgery and Oncology*, 3rd edn. (2003), p. 269.)

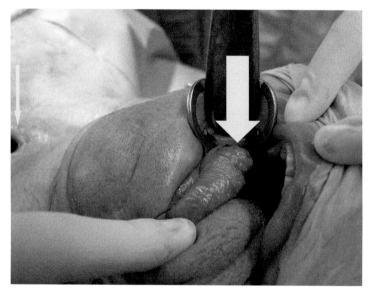

Fig. 1.9. Exophytic tongue tumor (large arrow) as a second primary tumor in a laryngectomized patient. Small arrow points to tracheostoma following total laryngectomy. Color version in plate section.

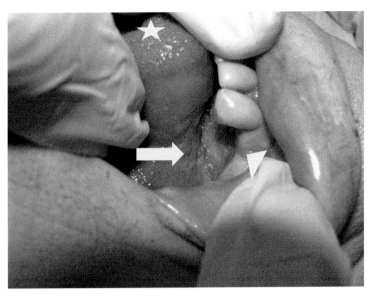

Fig. 1.10. Endophytic squamous cell carcinoma of the anterior floor of mouth (arrow) severely impairs tongue mobility as displayed by this attempt to move the tongue tip (yellow star) during the examination under general anesthesia (inferior alveolar ridge, arrowhead). At this time, the tumor is very far extended submucosally with only limited effect on speech and swallowing. Such extent can only be assessed correctly using radiological imaging. Color version in plate section.

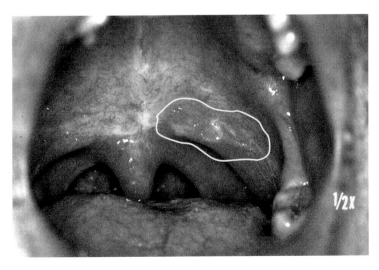

Fig. 1.11. Small recurrent oropharyngeal carcinoma on the soft palate (encircled by yellow line), 1 year following radiotherapy for a T2 N0 squamous cell carcinoma of the soft palate crossing the midline. Local pain and referred otalgia were the presenting symptoms of the recurrent lesion. Color version in plate section.

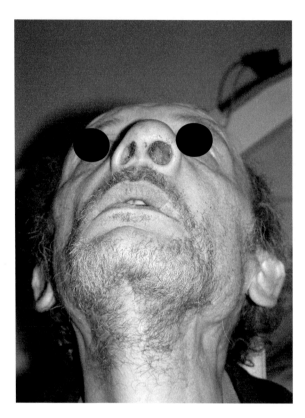

Fig. 1.12. Nasal obstruction brings this patient with squamous cell carcinoma of the nasal vestibule to the doctor. Color version in plate section.

symptoms caused by invasion of structures beyond the nasal cavity. Brain invasion through the anterior skull usually occurs late in the disease process.

Maxillary sinus cancer can cause trismus by invasion of the pterygoid muscles upon posterior extension, and palatal or alveolar ridge swelling upon downward extension; in the edentulous patient, failing denture fitting can be the first symptom (Fig. 1.13). Upward extension of maxillary SCC and lateral extension of ethmoidal SCC can cause orbital symptoms, mainly diplopia caused by prooptosis, but also caused by direct muscular invasion of the orbital muscles. Diplopia can also be caused by extension of SCC through the sphenoidal sinus to the cavernous sinus and invasion of the sixth and later third and fourth cranial nerves.

Such oculomotor paralysis can also be observed in advanced *nasopharyngeal* carcinoma extending to the skull base. A typical presentation of patients with nasopharyngeal carcinoma is unilateral serous otitis from Eustachian tube invasion and dysfunction. Otalgia is often associated with this pattern of spread. Most patients with nasopharyngeal cancer, however, are asymptomatic but present

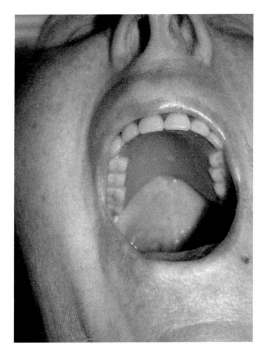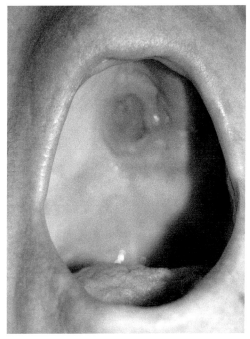

Fig. 1.13. Failing denture fitting in the upper jaw can be the first symptom of both oral cavity and maxillary sinus cancer. Color version in plate section.

with lymph node metastases, often extensive. In every level of the T classification of nasopharyngeal carcinoma, approximately four in five patients have clinical N2 or N3 disease at presentation [27].

Neck disease is, therefore, a frequent finding at presentation of patients with SCC arising at all sites of the head and neck. Following clinical examination and imaging, this regional tumor extent is adequately summarized in the N classification of the UICC TNM classification, which is true for all HNSCC with the exception of nasopharyngeal carcinoma [24]. For that subgroup, the massive neck nodal metastasis at presentation combined with the relatively good prognosis has resulted in a system where advanced neck disease results in a comparatively lower N classification (see also Chs. 6 and 7).

Clinical aspects of follow-up after diagnosis and successful treatment of malignant disease

Clinical follow-up after successful treatment of malignant HNSCC follows a rather rigid scheme of rigorous clinical examination intended to detect tumor recurrence in the treated area (Fig. 1.11) and in the neck, as well as new tumors (metachronous second primary tumors) in the rest of the upper aerodigestive tract (Fig. 1.9). Especially in index tumors treated radiotherapeutically, recurrences and second primaries are more difficult to detect because of radiation-induced tissue changes.

The annual incidence of second primary cancer following successful treatment of an index SCC in the head and neck area is 3–7%. A known feature in HNSCC is the observation of field cancerization of the upper aerodigestive tract: several synchronous and also metachronous primary carcinomas and areas of moderate to severe dysplasia – carcinoma in situ – are observed, with areas of normal mucous membranes between. This is caused by exposure of the entire upper aerodigestive tract to the same carcinogens – usually alcohol and tobacco. Patients are particularly at risk of developing lung cancer, esophageal and gastric cancer, and a new HNSCC. As already discussed under "risk factors", a change of lifestyle is essential to decrease the incidence of second primaries, but this is often difficult to achieve given the social context of the patient.

Conclusions

Head and neck SCC arises in the mucous membranes of the upper aerodigestive tract. This pathologically homogeneous disease presents in a very heterogeneous manner depending on the anatomical site of origin within the head and neck. Known risk factors have a different effect on different anatomical sites, and once a carcinoma develops, the clinical picture, the extent at diagnosis and thus the prognosis following treatment, also depend on the site of origin. This explains the site-specific approach in the chapters to follow.

ACKNOWLEDGEMENTS

The author would like to express his sincere gratitude to Pierre Delaere for providing Fig. 1.6 and Raf Sciot for providing the illustrative microscopic images (Figs. 1.4 and 1.5).

REFERENCES

1. R. T. Greenlee, M. B. Hill-Harmon, T. Murray, M. Thun. Cancer statistics, 2001. *CA Cancer J Clin* **51** (2001), 15–36.

2. D. M. Parkin, P. Pisani, J. Ferlay. Global cancer statistics. *CA Cancer J Clin* **49** (1999), 33–64.

3. International Agency for Research on Cancer. *Cancer Base 4. EUCAN: Cancer Incidence, Mortality and Prevalence in the European Union 1997*, version 4.0 (Lyon: IARC Press, 1999).

4. Vlaams Kankerregistratie Netwerk. *Kankerincidentie in Vlaanderen 1997–1999* (Brussels: Vlaamse Liga tegen Kanker VLK, 2002).

5. P. Boffetta, D. Trichopoulos. Cancer of the lung, larynx and pleura. In *Textbook of Cancer Epidemiology* (Oxford: Oxford University Press, 2002), pp. 268–72.

6. International Agency for Research on Cancer. *Cancer Incidence in Five Continents*, vol. VII (*Scientific Publication*, No. 143, ed. D. M. Parkin, S. L. Whelan, J. Ferley, *et al.*) Lyon: IARC Press, 1997), pp. i–xxxiv,1–1240.

7. G. L. Day, W. J. Blot, D. F. Austin, *et al.* Racial differences in risk of oral and pharyngeal cancer: alcohol, tobacco, and other determinants. *J Natl Cancer Inst* **85** (1993), 465–473.

8. D. P. De Rienzo, S. D. Greenberg, A. E. Fraire. Carcinoma of the larynx. Changing incidence in women. *Arch Otolaryngol Head Neck Surg* **117** (1991), 681–684.

9. W. J. Blot, J. K. McLaughlin, D. M. Winn, *et al.* Smoking and drinking in relation to oral and pharyngeal cancer. *Cancer Res* **48** (1988), 3282–3287.

10. D. E. Morse, R. V. Katz, D. G. Pendrys, *et al.* Smoking and drinking in relation to oral epithelial dysplasia. *Cancer Epidemiol Biomarkers Prev* **5** (1996), 769–777.

11. J. Brugere, P. Guenel, A. Leclerc, J. Rodriguez. Differential effects of tobacco and alcohol in cancer of the larynx, pharynx, and mouth. *Cancer* **57** (1986), 391–395.

12. E. De Stefani, A. Ronco, M. Mendilaharsu, H. Deneo-Pellegrini. Diet and risk of cancer of the upper aerodigestive tract: II. Nutrients. *Oral Oncol* **35** (1999), 22–26.

13. C. La Vecchia, A. Tavani, S. Franceschi, *et al.* Epidemiology and prevention of oral cancer. *Oral Oncol* **33** (1997), 302–312.

14. S. Franceschi, N. Munoz, X. F. Bosch, P. J. Snijders, J. M. Walboomers. Human papillomavirus and cancers of the upper aerodigestive tract: a review of epidemiological and experimental evidence. *Cancer Epidemiol Biomarkers Prev* **5** (1996), 567–575.

15. J. Lefebvre, E. Lartigau, A. Kara, J. Sarini. Oral cavity, pharynx and larynx cancer. Environment-related prognostic factors. In *UICC Prognostic Factors in Cancer* 2nd edn, ed. M. K. Gospodarowicz, D. E. Henson, R. V. P. Hutter, *et al.*, (New York: Wiley-Liss, 2001), pp. 151–165.

16. G. D'Souza, A. R. Kreimer, R. Viscidi, *et al.* Case–control study of human papillomavirus and oropharyngeal cancer. *N Engl J Med* **356** (2007), 1944–1956.

17. D. Jeannel, G. Bouvier, A. Hubert. Nasopharyngeal cancer. In *Infections and Human Cancer*, ed. R. Newton, V. Beral, R. A. Weiss (New York: Cold Spring Harbor Press, 1999), pp. 125–156.

18. E. Pedersen, A. C. Hogetveit, A. Andersen. Cancer of respiratory organs among workers at nickel refinery in Norway. *Int J Cancer* **12** (1973), 32–41.

19. World Health Organization Collaborating Centre for Oral Precancerous Lesions. Definitions of leukoplakia and related lesions: an aid to studies on oral precancer. *Oral Surg Oral Med Oral Pathol* **46** (1978), 518–539.

20. J. G. Batsakis. Clinical pathology of oral cancer. In *Oral Cancer*, ed. J. P. Shah, N. W. Johnson, J. G. Batsakis. (London: Martin Dunitz, Taylor and Francis Group, 2003), pp. 77–129.

21. S. J. Silverman, M. Gorsky, G. E. Kaugars. Leukoplakia, dysplasia, and malignant transformation. *Oral Surg Oral Med Oral Pathol* **82** (1996), 117.

22. J. E. Medina, W. Dichtel, M. A. Luna. Verrucous-squamous carcinomas of the oral cavity. A clinicopathologic study of 104 cases. *Arch Otolaryngol* **110** (1984), 437–440.

23. J. P. Shah. Patterns of cervical lymph node metastasis from squamous carcinomas of the upper aerodigestive tract. *Am J Surg* **160** (1990), 405–409.

24. L. H. Sobin, C. Wittekind (eds.) *UICC TNM Classification of Malignant Tumors,* 6th edn (New York: Wiley-Liss, 2002), pp. 30–31.

25. W. M. Lydiatt, D. D. Lydiatt. The larynx: early stage disease. In *Cancer of the Head and Neck*, ed. J. P. Shah (London: BC Decker, 2001), pp. 169–184.

26. J. P. Shah. Larynx and trachea. In *Head and Neck Surgery and Oncology*, ed. J. P. Shah, S. G. Patel, 3rd edn (New York: Mosby, 2003), pp. 269–352.

27. R. Lindberg. Distribution of cervical lymph node metastases from squamous cell carcinoma of the upper respiratory and digestive tracts. *Cancer* **29** (1972), 1446–1449.

2

Radiotherapy and chemoradiotherapy of the head and neck

Sandra Nuyts

Introduction

Radiation oncology plays a major role in the treatment of cancers of the head and neck. It can be used as the only treatment modality or as an adjuvant treatment in combination with surgery. In recent years, it has been frequently used in combination with chemotherapy, mainly to preserve organ function.

In the last decades, important advances in the delivery of radiotherapy have been made, making it possible to deliver high doses of radiation to the tumor, while maximally sparing the surrounding tissues. These developments imply, however, a very accurate delineation of the tumor-involved tissues, which can only be made via the use of imaging techniques.

(Chemo)radiotherapy in head and neck cancer

Selection of a treatment modality

Selection of a treatment modality for head and neck cancer should be based on the size and location of the primary tumor, the status of the regional lymph nodes and the general condition of the patient. Early head and neck cancers are usually treated with one modality – either surgery or radiation therapy. The choice between surgery and radiation therapy in these cases is usually determined by the functional deficit that would result from each treatment modality, since both result in similar rates of local control and survival. Cancers at a locally advanced stage can be treated with a combination of surgery and (chemo)radiotherapy or with primary (chemo)radiotherapy. Chemoradiotherapy can be used when organ preservation is feasible, with surgery as an optional salvage treatment. This benefit is most clearly established in laryngeal cancer but is increasingly recognized for other anatomic locations [1].

Squamous Cell Cancer of the Neck, ed. Robert Hermans. Published by Cambridge University Press.
© R. Hermans 2009.

Radiation therapy alone

Most primary radiotherapy is delivered through external beam irradiation. Radiation portals encompass the macroscopic tumor and possible microscopic extension and the pathologically involved lymph nodes. Elective lymph node regions are irradiated if a risk greater than 15% of subclinical metastasis exists in these areas.

The tumor dose is usually based on the extent of the cancer and the tolerance of normal tissues in the treated area. In case of limited disease, doses of 60 to 65 Gy in 6 to 6.5 weeks may be adequate. Higher doses (e.g., 65–75 Gy in 6.5 to 7.5 weeks) are needed for larger tumors. Using conventional fractionation, patients receive one radiotherapy session per day, five per week, during 6 to 7 weeks. Based on radiobiological insights, radiotherapy with altered fractionation is being increasingly adopted, also in patients with early disease since it may offer a better outcome than after conventional fractionation [2,3]. Treating the patients, for example, twice daily or with six fractions a week, offers the possibility of reducing the overall treatment time and/or increasing the dose to the tumor, leading to increased tumor control.

The treatment is usually delivered with a shrinking-field technique (Fig. 2.1). An initial dose of 45 to 50 Gy is delivered in 4 to 5 weeks through large portals covering the clinically involved region and areas of potential regional lymph node metastasis. Thereafter, the fields are reduced to encompass only the gross tumor with a smaller margin, and an additional dose of 15 to 25 Gy is delivered, bringing the total tumor dose to 60 to 75 Gy in 6 to 7.5 weeks. To avoid the risk of radiation myelitis, the dose to the spinal cord is kept below 45 to 50 Gy.

Combined surgery and radiation therapy

Although no large randomized trial has been carried out, postoperative radiotherapy has become the standard in many institutions, especially for stage III–IV tumors (Table 2.1). Radiation therapy is used to eradicate microscopic extensions of tumors that cannot be excised and preferably starts within 6 weeks after surgery.

High-risk indications for postoperative radiotherapy are microscopically involved resection margins and/or extracapsular extension of nodal disease [4,5].

Intermediate risk indications for adjuvant radiotherapy are

close resection margins < 5 mm

pathological lymph node involvement in two or more nodes

T3 or T4 tumors

perineural involvement

oral cavity tumors.

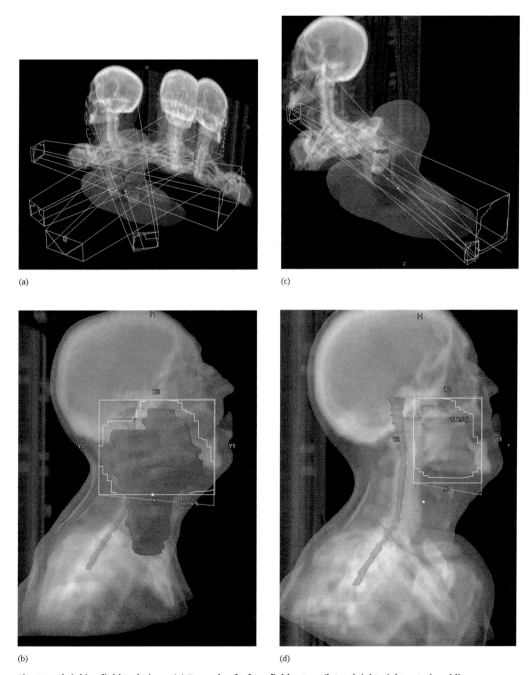

(a)

(c)

(b)

(d)

Fig. 2.1. Shrinking field technique. (a) Example of a four-field set-up (lateral right, right anterior oblique, left anterior oblique and lower anterior field) for a patient with a tumor in the right paralingual sulcus. Radiation portals encompass the tumoral volumes and all elective lymph node regions (in red). **(b)** The lateral right large radiation field. **(c)** After a dose of 45–50 Gy, radiation portals are shrunk so that they only encompass the tumor-involved tissues (in yellow) and spare the spinal cord (in pink). **(d)** The right posterior oblique field. These so-called boost fields (c,d) deliver the additional boost dose to the demonstrable gross tumor. Color version in plate section.

Table 2.1. Stage grouping of head and neck tumors

	N0	N1	N2a	N2b	N2c	N3
T1	Stage I	Stage III	Stage IVa	Stage IVa	Stage IVa	Stage IVb
T2	Stage II	Stage III	Stage IVa	Stage IVa	Stage IVa	Stage IVb
T3	Stage III	Stage III	Stage IVa	Stage IVa	Stage IVa	Stage IVb
T4	Stage IVa	Stage IVa	Stage IVa	Stage IVa	Stage IVa	Stage IVb

Even with adjuvant radiotherapy in the presence of high-risk features, the risk of local recurrence (27–61%), distant metastasis (18–21%) and death (5-year survival rate 27–34%) remains unsatisfactorily high. The role of altered fractionation in this population is, therefore, under investigation.

The role of chemoradiotherapy in these patient groups has been examined by two large randomized trials by the European Organization for Research and Treatment of Cancer (EORTC) and the Radiation Therapy Oncology Group (RTOG) [6,7]. Both trials used concomitant cisplatin every 3 weeks during the course of radiotherapy (60–66 Gy) and demonstrated that adjuvant concurrent chemoradiotherapy was more efficient than radiotherapy alone in terms of local control and disease-free survival in high-risk patients. Only in the EORTC trial was overall survival significantly increased with chemoradiotherapy. Surprisingly, no impact on distant metastases was seen in both trials. The gain in local control, however, implied a significant increase in incidence of severe acute adverse events. Further clinical research is needed to improve outcome in patients with high risk of failure after surgery.

Chemoradiotherapy

Since the mid to late 1990s, chemoradiotherapy has been shown to improve markedly both survival and organ preservation. A large meta-analysis from the Meta-analysis of Chemotherapy in Head and Neck Cancer (MACH-NC) collaborative group showed an absolute survival benefit of 8% at 5 years for concurrent chemoradiotherapy [8,9]. The largest benefit was seen with platinum-based chemotherapy, and no significant difference was seen between mono- or polychemotherapy. Concurrent chemoradiotherapy with further surgery reserved for salvage offers the potential for larynx preservation without compromising survival in advanced disease of the larynx or hypopharynx. The benefit of chemoradiotherapy must be weighed against the toxicity inherent in its use. The risk of acute mucositis, dermatitis and chemotherapy-specific side effects is greater than with either mode of therapy alone. Short-term use of gastric feeding devices is needed more frequently. In those studies that have assessed long-term function, no increase in long-term toxicities was noted. The latest generation of studies continues to show improved survival rates when chemotherapy is added to hyperfractionated radiotherapy [3].

The probability of distant metastases remains high after concurrent chemo-radiotherapy (15–20% at 5 years), indicating a lesser than expected role of chemother-apy in reducing distant spread.

The role of induction chemotherapy followed by definitive local therapy is currently the subject of intense debate. The MACH-NC meta-analyses showed no benefit in the use of induction chemotherapy (usually cisplatin and 5-fluorouracil [PF]) [8,9]. However, the introduction of taxanes in induction chemotherapy regi-mens (cisplatin plus 5-fluorouracil plus a taxane [TPF]) has shown superiority in comparison with older PF schedules in three recent trials [10–12]. Still, induction chemotherapy cannot be considered as standard therapy, since no direct comparison has been made between induction chemotherapy and concurrent chemoradiother-apy. The results of these trials are still awaited.

Novel targeted therapies

The majority of HNSCC has increased levels of epidermal growth factor receptor (EGFR) production, which has been correlated with disease progression. Many studies have also shown that EGFR overproduction can be an adverse prognostic factor for cancer treatment outcome, making it an interesting target for new therapies. Cetuximab is a mouse–human chimeric antibody that binds to EGFR and blocks binding of EGF and transforming growth factor alpha to the receptor. This inhibits activation of the EGFR tyrosine kinase. A recent published phase III trial randomized patients with locally advanced head and neck cancer between radio-therapy alone versus radiotherapy and concurrent weekly cetuximab [13]. The addition of cetuximab showed an absolute improvement in local control and overall survival at 2 years of 8% and 13%, respectively. These gains, which are comparable to the gains attained by adding chemotherapy to radiotherapy, were accomplished without increase in acute toxicity. Despite the clear positive results of this study, the role of cetuximab today is still unclear since the control arm in the study is considered inferior in the light of current information. Trials are ongoing exploring the role of cetuximab and other targeted agents in comparison with chemoradiotherapy.

Toxicity and complications of chemoradiotherapy

The benefit of chemoradiotherapy must be weighed against the toxicity inherent in its use. The risk of acute mucositis, dermatitis and chemotherapy-specific side effects is greater than with either mode of therapy alone. The increase of acute, especially mucosal, toxicity often necessitates feeding-tube placement. The effect on late toxicity has yet to be elucidated. The side effects with the highest impact on the quality of life are speech and swallowing changes. To decrease the risk of long-term side effects, preventative measures are suggested, such as avoiding radiotherapy to the pharyngeal musculature, speech-language pathologist evaluation throughout the course of therapy with swallowing exercises and delay in feeding tube placement as long as possible.

Given the toxicity of chemoradiotherapy, careful selection of patients is critical. Many issues remain to be addressed in future trials, including the optimal chemotherapy regimen, the use of altered fractionation radiotherapy and the role of induction chemotherapy.

Imaging needs in conformal radiation therapy

Radiotherapy, as a cornerstone in treatment of head and neck cancer, has undergone substantial improvements. While, until the early 1990s, treatment portals were based on two-dimensional radiographic simulation film, introduction of computed tomography (CT) allows us now to design radiation portals in the shape of the tumor in three dimensions, so-called three-dimensional conformal radiotherapy (3D-CRT) (Fig. 2.2). Recent improvements in computer technology have also led to the development of better techniques for delivering a high dose of radiation to the target volumes and a smaller dose to normal tissues, leading to an increased therapeutic gain. Such techniques are called conformal because the high-dose region is designed to conform to the target volume. At the same time, advancements in diagnostic imaging have made it possible to define better the extent of the cancer. These two advances are complementary, leading to a powerful new tool for the management of many head and neck cancers.

Intensity-modulated radiation therapy (IMRT) is one method of delivering conformal radiation therapy. As its name implies, IMRT allows the intensity of each radiation beam to be modulated, so that each field may have one or more areas of high-intensity radiation, while other areas receive lower doses. By modulating the number of fields and the intensity within each field, radiation dose can be sculpted around the tumor. The radiation oncologist outlines various tumor

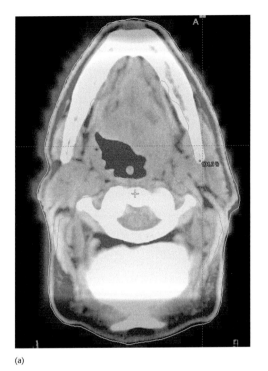

(a)

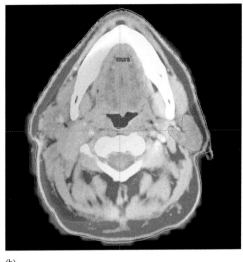

(b)

Fig. 2.2. Two- and three-dimensional radiotherapy. (a) In two-dimensional radiotherapy, radiation portals are designed on routine simulation films to encompass the desired target volume. The resulting isodoses show good coverage of the target volumes (contoured in red), but poor sparing of normal tissues, for example the parotid gland (colorwash isodoses: red, high-dose region; blue–green, low-dose region). (b) In three-dimensional conformal radiotherapy, precision radiotherapy offers the possibility for reducing the dose to normal tissues. In this patient with a tumor in the tonsillar area, a four-field set-up was arranged, allowing good sparing of the controlateral parotid gland, as shown in the isodoses. Color version in plate section.

volumes (e.g., primary tumor, nodal disease, subclinical volumes) on treatment-planning CT scans, along with critical organs and normal structures (Fig. 2.3). Each structure is assigned a target dose and an acceptable range of doses. The computer considers these dosage limits as it develops a treatment-delivery plan.

Crucial in this process is, of course, the accurate delineation of target volumes and organs at risk. Since with IMRT the radiation dose is sculpted around the tumor, the risk of marginal misses becomes evident if the exact tumor extension is not taken into account. Imaging methods have, therefore, become used more and more in defining radiation portals. Both anatomical imaging and functional imaging have gained status in helping the radiation oncologist define the target. Also during the course of radiotherapy, imaging methods are being used more and more for treatment verification and adaptation.

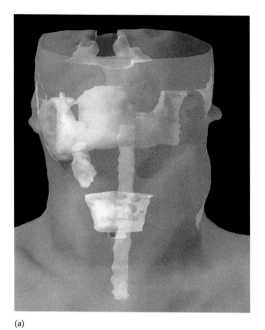
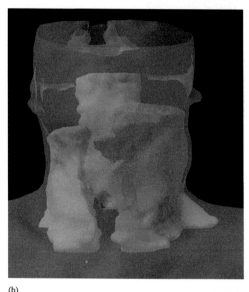

(a)   (b)

Fig. 2.3. Computed tomograph allows the radiation oncologist to contour on each slice the gross tumor volumes and the relevant organs at risk. (a) Three-dimensional reconstructions can be generated, representing the organs at risk (e.g., the parotid glands in green and blue, the mandible in light red, spinal cord in pink, larynx in yellow, submandibular glands in light green and dark blue, and brainstem in brown). (b) The target volumes of the same patient; the elective lymph node regions are contoured in orange, while the tumor in the piriform sinus and the involved nodes are depicted in red. Color version in plate section.

Use of imaging modalities in defining the target

Anatomical information

At present, CT is used for initial delineation of tumor volumes and is considered the gold standard. Before the start of radiotherapy, patients receive a CT scan, preferably with intravenous contrast, in treatment position. To assure accurate positioning during the course of radiotherapy, patients are immobilized using a thermoplastic mask (Fig. 2.4). The dataset is transferred to a planning computer and the radiation oncologist contours the tumoral and relevant normal tissues on each CT slice, with a thickness of preferably 3 to 5 mm (Fig. 2.5). As the image quality of such a study is less good than can be achieved on a diagnostic CT study, the latter is correlated with the planning scan. Around the macroscopic tumor (so-called gross tumor volume [GTV]) a margin is added to take account of the microscopic extension of the tumor (so-called clinical target volume [CTV]). To account for small variations in positioning of the patient and/or movement of the tumor, an additional margin is added, resulting in the so-called planning target

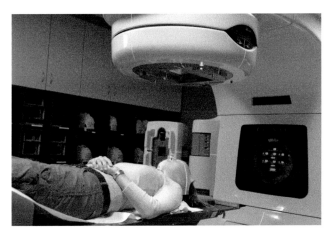

Fig. 2.4. To allow accurate and reproducible immobilization during a course of 6–7 weeks of radiotherapy, patients are immobilized using a thermoplastic mask. Color version in plate section.

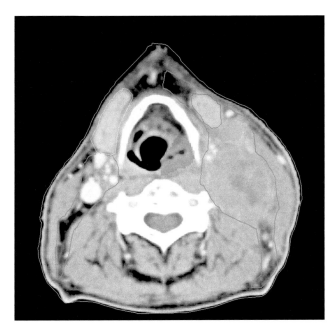

Fig. 2.5. On each CT slice, the radiation oncologist contours relevant structures. The primary tumor in the piriform sinus is contoured in shaded red, the pathologically involved lymph nodes in shaded orange. Elective lymph node regions to be irradiated are contoured in red. Both submandibular glands and the spinal cord are contoured on this slide as organs at risk. Color version in plate section.

volume (PTV). Based on these contours, radiation portals are defined and a treatment plan is generated to ascertain the planned dose is delivered to the PTV. Therefore, the electron densities as shown on CT are used in the planning system for dose calculation. However, for some patients, CT is not sufficient for excellent tumor delineation. Certainly for nasopharyngeal cancer and base of tongue tumors, magnetic resonance imaging (MRI) can deliver complementary information. Enami *et al.* examined the use of CT and MRI in eight patients with nasopharyngeal cancer [14]. Compared with CT, the MRI-based targets were 74% larger, more irregularly shaped and did not always include the CTV targets. Chung *et al.* (2004) confirmed this in a study of 258 patients [15]. Their study showed that MRI was superior for detection of intracranial infiltration since in 40.3% of patients this was detected on MRI when CT showed negative findings. Also detection of pterygopalatine fossa involvement was higher with MRI than CT (96.1% versus 56.9%). Image fusion of both CT and MRI allows one to use both CT and MRI information in drawing the target volumes (Fig. 2.6).

Functional/biological information

The use of positron emission tomography (PET) in target delineation for head and neck cancer is under investigation. The use of PET with 2-[F-18]-fluoro-2-deoxy-D-glucose (^{18}F-fluorodeoxyglucose [FDG]) particularly when combined can help in defining tumoral tissues with CT. However one crucial comment must be made concerning the interpretation of PET images. If PET is used to delineate volumes, the way the PET images are viewed must be defined. For example, changing the window setting changes the interpretation of lesion margins; the optimal window setting for radiotherapy contouring applications has yet to be determined. Until now, every study uses its own threshold, or does not comment on which threshold was used, which makes it difficult to compare the data. Several studies have investigated the influence and accuracy of FDG PET in target volume definition as a complementary study to CT. Radiotherapy volumes were altered and the GTV measured by PET was increased in some patients compared with that delineated by CT, while in others it was reduced. It was concluded that PET can act as a complementary modality, providing information on target viability that was not visible by CT [16–20]. These authors, therefore, recommend using both CT- and PET-defined primary tumor in determining the GTV for IMRT.

In addition to FDG, other tracers are being investigated. These tracers may give an insight into the biological features of the tumor and ideally predict the response of the tumor to a certain therapy. Tracers depicting hypoxia are of particular interest since hypoxia is believed to be a major determinant in tumor response to radiation. If these resistant regions within the tumor can be delineated, dose escalation to those parts could be performed, potentially increasing local control (Fig. 2.7). Several tracers are under development and some are being tested in clinical studies. Tracers such as ^{18}F-misonidazole have already been shown to predict poorer outcome to radiotherapy when high levels of uptake occur [21]. The marker ^{62}Cu-diacetylbis(N-4-methyl-thiosemicaarbazone [Cu-ATSM]) is a potentially good marker for hypoxia because of its rapid uptake, activity ratio, rapid blood clearance and washout from normally oxygenated cells. Chao *et al.* (2001) examined the feasibility

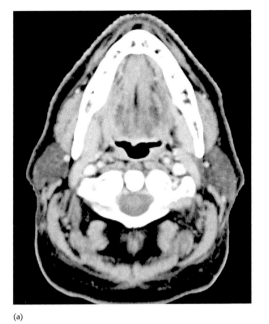

(a)

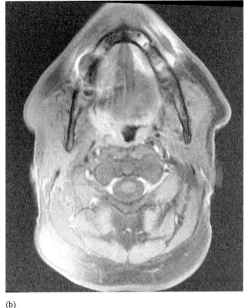

(b)

(c)

Fig. 2.6. The use of MRI in combination with CT to allow accurate delineation of a tumor. (a) The CT scan of a patient with a squamous cell carcinoma in the right lateral oropharyngeal wall, extending to the glossotonsillar sulcus and base of tongue. (b) The corresponding gadolinium-enhanced T_1-weighted spin-echo MRI image. (c) This can be co-registered with the CT by the planning software, allowing contouring on both CT and MRI.

of dose escalation to hypoxic areas using IMRT by co-registration of Cu-ATSM PET with CT images for treatment planning [22]. This planning study showed that 80 Gy could be delivered in 35 fractions to the hypoxic target volume, with 70 Gy in 35 fractions delivered to the rest of the clinical target volume.

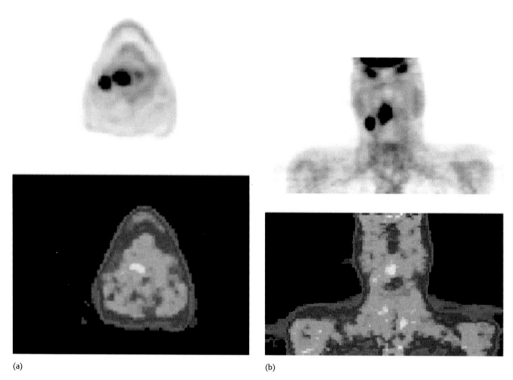

(a)   (b)

Fig. 2.7. Position emission tomography (PET) of tumors. (a) A ^{18}F-fluorodeoxyglucose scan of a patient with a T3 N1 squamous cell carcinoma of the right tonsil. Both tumor and involved lymph node can be visualized on the axial and coronal plane. (b) The corresponding scan using ^{18}F-misonidazole for the same patient. Some parts of both the primary tumor and the enlarged lymph node show high uptake of tracer (bright green), suggesting the presence of hypoxia in these regions. Color version in plate section.

As with PET, the use of functional MRI in radiotherapy planning is a field of intense research. Several MRI techniques can help to characterize the biological target volume: perfusion MRI (angiogenesis), MR spectroscopy (metabolism), diffusion-weighted MRI (cellularity) and Four-dimension MRI (4D-MRI; motion) [reviewed by Khoo and Joon 23]. Again, if these imaging modalities can define regions within the tumor that are more resistant to radiotherapy, based on the biological information gained, dose-escalation can be performed to these subdomains.

Use of imaging modalities in treatment verification and adaptation

Radiotherapy for head and neck cancer typically spans 6 to 7 weeks. During this time, many anatomical changes can occur. Patients can lose weight, tumor shrinkage occurs or edema develops, all leading to shifting of tumoral and normal tissue

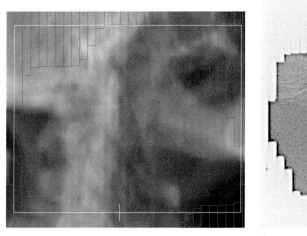
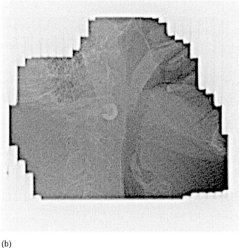

(a)   (b)

Fig. 2.8. Treatment verification can be performed using portal images. (a) The expected treatment field is shown by the digitally reconstructed radiograph, based on CT images. (b) The actual treatment field is presented by the portal image, taken during irradiation. Both images are compared to verify positioning of the patient, and size and shape of the treatment portal.

positions. Treatment guiding and verification refers to the use of imaging to ensure that the field of irradiation is appropriate throughout the entire treatment period, taking into consideration factors such as changes in tumor size and shape, patient positioning and organ movement. Today, the treatment fields are routinely verified using the accelerator beam and conventional film or, in modern systems, using two-dimensional electronic portal image detectors (EPID; Fig. 2.8). Recently, cone-beam CT has been introduced for verification of treatment fields, allowing a three-dimensional visualization of the treatment field in relation to organs of interest on the treatment machine (Fig. 2.9). Treatment can be adapted based on this information, leading to the so-called adaptive or image-guided radiotherapy. Strategies are being developed to adjust treatment plans in real time to account for differences in anatomy.

Conclusions

Improvements in radiotherapy techniques leading to very conformal dose distributions inherently imply very accurate delineation of tumoral and non-tumoral tissues. Until now, no single imaging modality allows us to appreciate the exact tumoral extension. Anatomical and functional imaging modalities will be complementary,

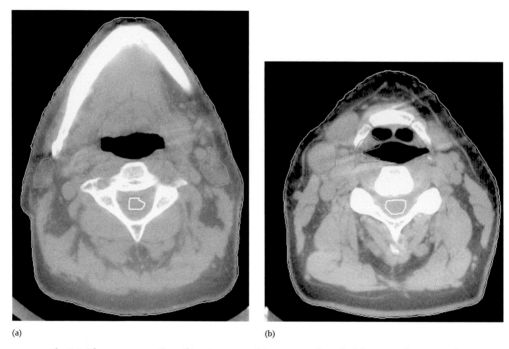

(a)   (b)

Fig. 2.9. The new generation of treatment machines are equipped with megavoltage cone-beam CT, allowing verification of patient/tumor positioning in real time. The images have sufficient quality to allow contouring of organs at risk (a) and tumor-involved tissues (b). Color version in plate section.

and fusion of these images will be necessary. In future, imaging during radiotherapy will allow us to correct the treatment plan according to anatomical and hopefully biological information, leading to adaptive radiotherapy.

REFERENCES

1. A. A. Forastiere, H. Goepfert, M. Maor, *et al.* Concurrent chemotherapy and radiotherapy for organ preservation in advanced laryngeal cancer. *N Engl J Med* **349** (2003), 2091–2098.
2. J. Bourhis, J. Overgaard, H. Audry, *et al.* for the Meta-Analysis of Radiotherapy in Carcinomas of Head and neck (MARCH) Collaborative Group. Hyperfractionated or accelerated radiotherapy in head and neck cancer: a meta-analysis. *Lancet*, **368** (2006), 843–584.
3. W. Budach, T. Hehr, V. Budach, C. Belka, K. Dietz. A meta-analysis of hyperfractionated and accelerated radiotherapy and combined chemotherapy regimens in unresected locally advanced squamous cell carcinoma of the head and neck. *BMC Cancer* **6** (2006), 28.

4. L. J. Peters, H. Goepfert, K. K. Ang, *et al.* Evaluation of the dose for postoperative radiation therapy of head and neck cancer: first report of a prospective randomized trial. *Int J Radiat Oncol Biol Phys* **26** (1993), 3–11.

5. K. K. Ang, A. Trotti, B. W. Brown, *et al.* Randomized trial addressing risk features and time factors of surgery plus radiotherapy in advanced head-and-neck cancer. *Int J Radiat Oncol Biol Phys* **51** (2001), 571–578.

6. J. Bernier, C. Domenge, M. Ozsahin, *et al.* European Organization for Research and Treatment of Cancer Trial 22931. Postoperative irradiation with or without concomitant chemotherapy for locally advanced head and neck cancer. *N Engl J Med* **350** (2004), 1945–1952.

7. J. S. Cooper, T. F. Pajak, A. A. Forastiere, *et al.* Postoperative concurrent radiotherapy and chemotherapy for high-risk squamous-cell carcinoma of the head and neck. *N Engl J Med* **350** (2004), 1937–1944.

8. J. P. Pignon, J. Bourhis, C. Domenge, L. Designe for the MACH-NC Collaborative Group. Chemotherapy added to locoregional treatment for head and neck squamous-cell carcinoma: three meta-analyses of updated individual data. *Lancet* **355** (2000), 949–955.

9. J. Bourhis, C. Amand, J.P. Pignon for the MACH-NC Collaborative Group. Update of the MACH-NC (meta-analysis of chemotherapy in head and neck cancer) database focused on concomitant chemoradiotherapy. *J Clin Oncol* **22** (2004), S5505.

10. M. R Posner, B. Glisson, G. Frenette, *et al.* Multicenter phase I–II trial of docetaxel, cisplatin, and fluorouracil induction chemotherapy for patients with locally advanced squamous cell cancer of the head and neck. *J Clin Oncol* **19** (2001), 1096–1104.

11. J. B. Vermorken, E. Remenar, C. Van Herpen, *et al.* Standard cisplatin/infusional 5-fluorouracil (PF) vs. docetaxel (T) plus PF (TPF) as neo-adjuvant chemotherapy for non-resectable locally advanced head and neck cancer (LAHNC): a phase III of the EORTC head and neck cancer group (EORTC 24971). *J Clin Oncol* **22** (2004), S5508.

12. R. Hitt, J. Grau, A. Lopez-Pousa, *et al.* Randomized phase II/III clinical trial of induction chemotherapy (ICT) with either cisplatin/5-fluorouracil (PF) or docetaxel/cisplatin/ 5-fluorouracil (TPF) followed by chemoradiotherapy (CRT) vs. CRT alone for patients with unresectable locally advanced head and neck cancer (LAHNC). *J Clin Oncol* **24** (2006), S5515.

13. J. A. Bonner, P. M. Harari, J. Giralt, *et al.* Radiotherapy plus cetuximab for squamous cell carcinoma of the head and neck. *N Engl J Med* **354** (2006), 567–578.

14. B. Enami, A. Sethi, G. J. Petruzelli. Influence of MRI on target volume delineation and IMRT planning in nasopharyngeal carcinoma. *Int J Radiat Oncol Biol Phys* **57** (2003), 481–488.

15. N. N. Chung, L. L. Ting, W. C. Hsu, L. T. Lui, P. M. Wang. Impact of magnetic resonance imaging versus CT on nasopharyngeal carcinoma: primary tumor target delineation for radiotherapy. *Head Neck* **26** (2004), 241–246.

16. C. Scarfone, W. C. Lavely, A. J. Cmelak, *et al.* Prospective feasibility trial of radiotherapy target definition for head and neck cancer using 3-dimensional PET and CT imaging. *J Nucl Med* **45** (2004), 543–552.

17. M. Koshy, A. C. Paulino, R. Howell, *et al.* F-18 FDG PET-CT fusion in radiotherapy treatment planning for head and neck cancer. *Head Neck* **27** (2005), 494–502.

18. A. C. Paulino, M. Koshy, R. Howell, D. Schuster, L. W. Davis. Comparison of CT- and FDG-PET-defined gross tumor volume in intensity-modulated radiotherapy for head-and-neck cancer. *Int J Radiat Oncol Biol Phys* **61** (2005), 1385–1392.

19. F. I. Ciernik, E. Dizendorf, B. Baumert, *et al.* Radiation treatment planning with an integrated positron emission and computer tomography (PET/CT): a feasibility study. *Int J Radiat Oncol Biol Phys* **57** (2003), 853–863.

20. T. Nishioka, T. Shiga, H. Shirato, *et al.* Image fusion between 18FDG-PET and MRI/CT for radiotherapy planning of oropharyngeal and nasopharyngeal carcinomas. *Int J Radiat Oncol Biol Phys* **53** (2002), 1051–1057.

21. D. Rischin, R. J. Hicks, R. Fisher, *et al.* for the Trans-Tasman Radiation Oncology Group Study 98.02. Prognostic significance of [18F]-misonidazole positron emission tomography-detected tumor hypoxia in patients with advanced head and neck cancer randomly assigned to chemo-radiation with or without tirapazamine: a substudy of Trans-Tasman Radiation Oncology Group Study 98.02. *J Clin Oncol* **24** (2006), 2098–2104.

22. C. Chao, W. R. Bosch, S. Mutic, *et al.* A novel approach to overcome hypoxic tumor resistance: Cu-ATSM-guided intensity-modulated radiation therapy. *Int J Radiat Oncol Biol Phys* **49** (2001), 1171–1182.

23. V. S. Khoo, D. L. Joon. New developments in MRI for target volume delineation in radiotherapy. *Br J Radiol* **79** (2006), S2–S15.

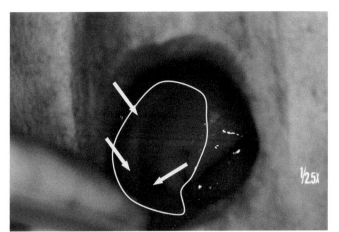

Fig. 1.2

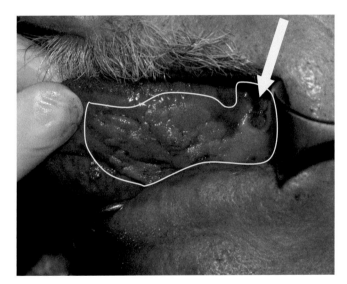

Fig. 1.3

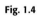

Fig. 1.4

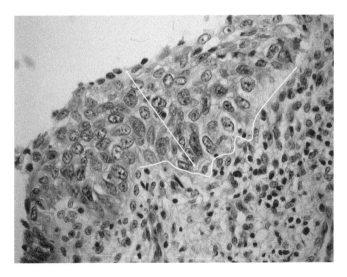

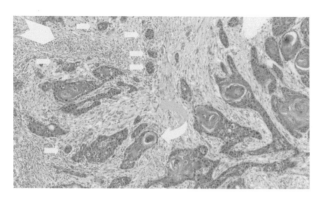

Fig. 1.5

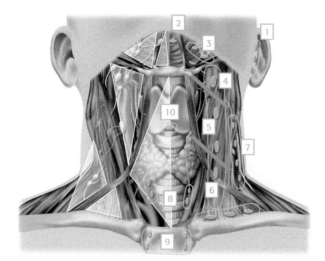

Fig. 1.6

Fig. 1.7

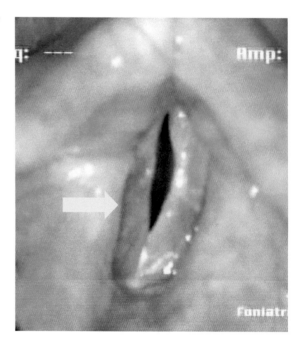

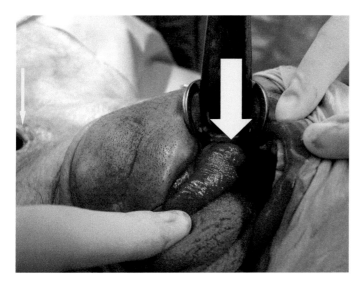

Fig. 1.9

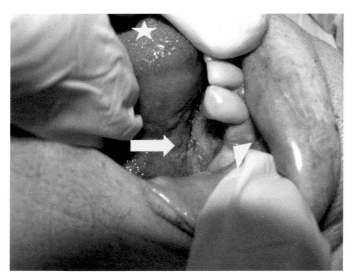

Fig. 1.10

Fig. 1.11

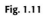

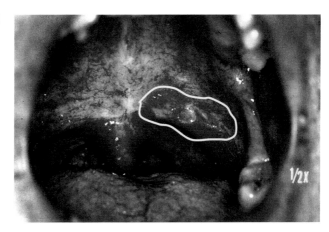

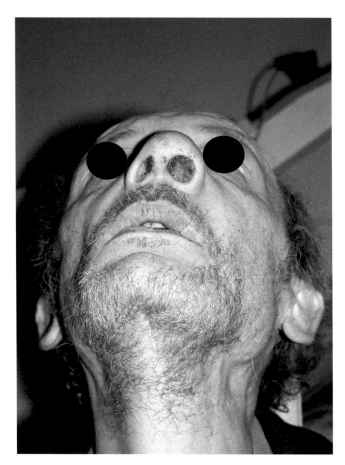

Fig. 1.12

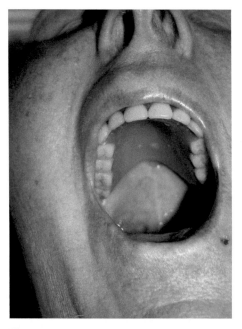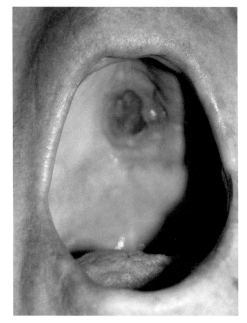

Fig. 1.13

Fig. 2.1a–d

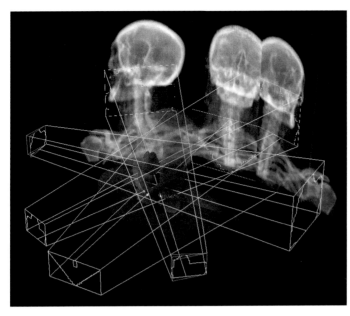

(a)

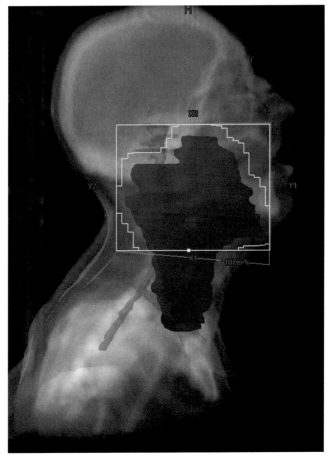

(b)

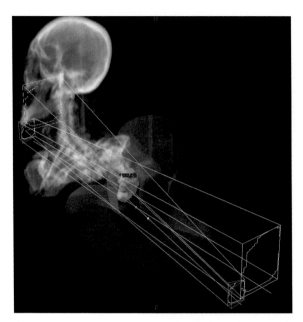

(c)

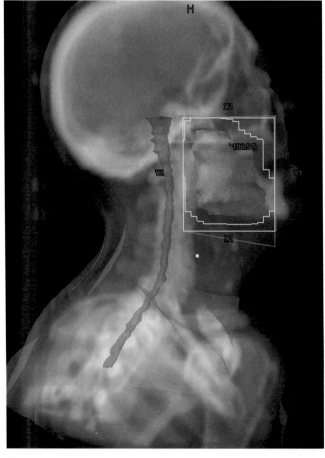

(d)

Fig. 2.1 (cont.)

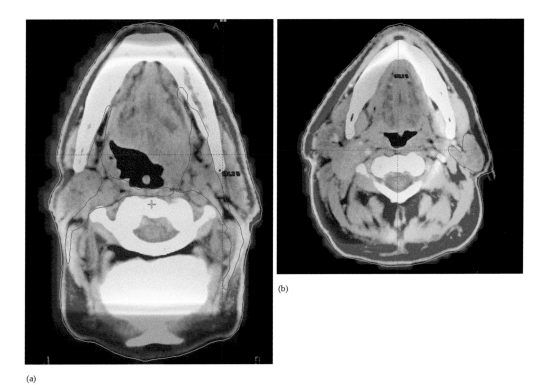

(a)

(b)

Fig. 2.2a,b

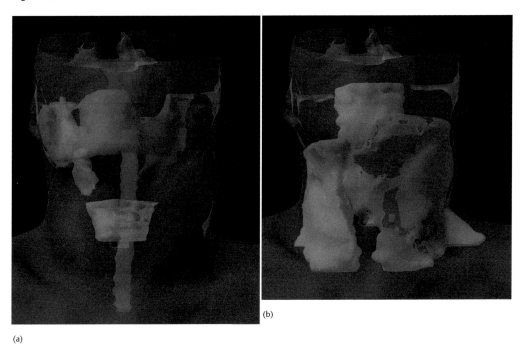

(a)

(b)

Fig. 2.3a,b

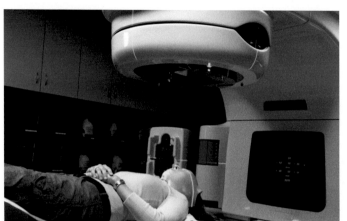

Fig. 2.4

Fig. 2.5

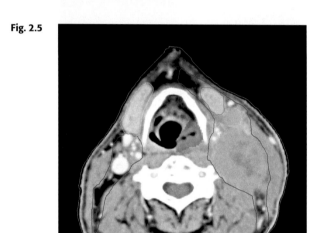

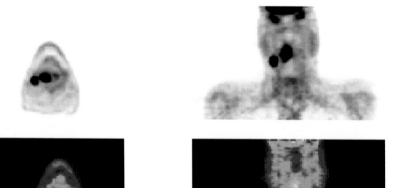

(a)

(b)

Fig. 2.7

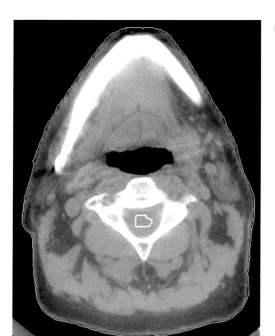

(a)

Fig. 2.9a,b

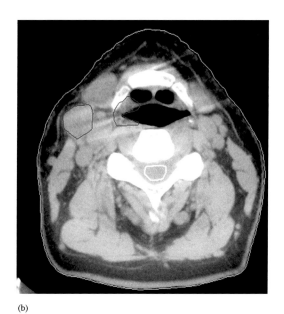

(b)

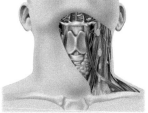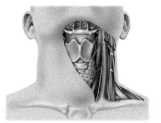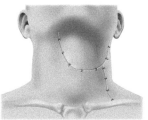

Fig. 3.1

Fig. 3.2

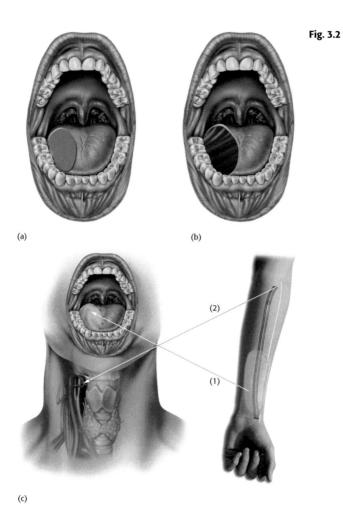

(a)

(b)

(c)

(2)

(1)

Fig. 3.3

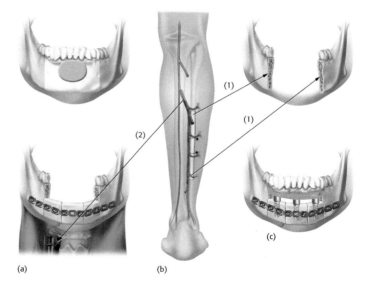

(1)

(1)

(2)

(a)

(b)

(c)

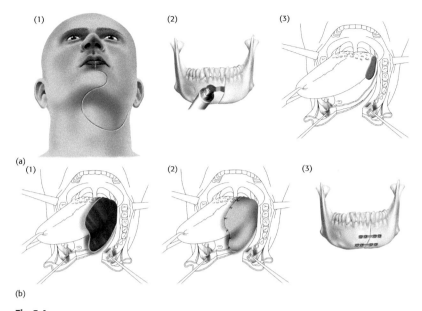

(a)

(b)

Fig. 3.4

Fig. 3.5

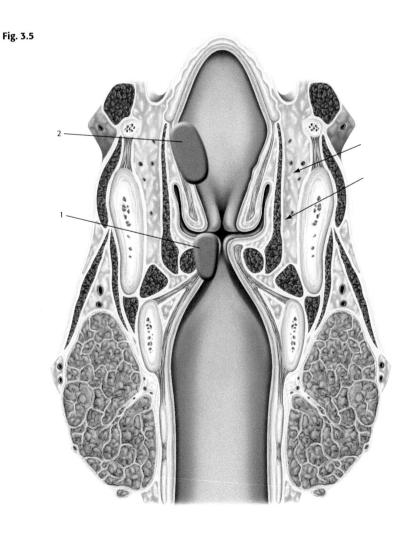

Fig. 3.6

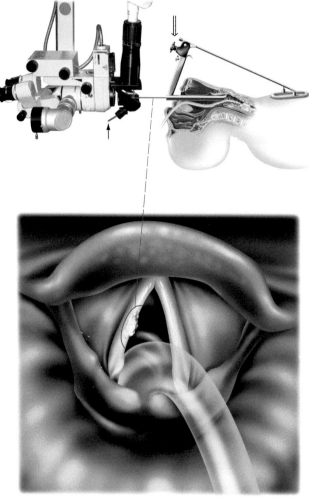

(a)

Fig. 3.7

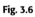

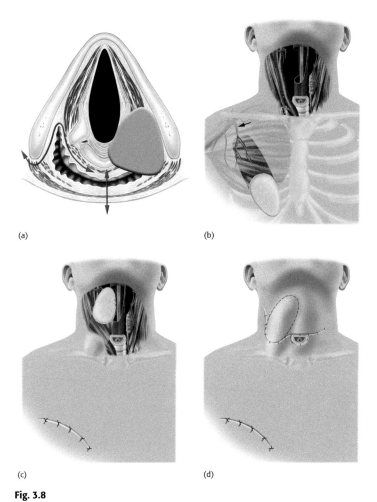

(a)

(b)

(c)

(d)

Fig. 3.8

Fig. 3.9

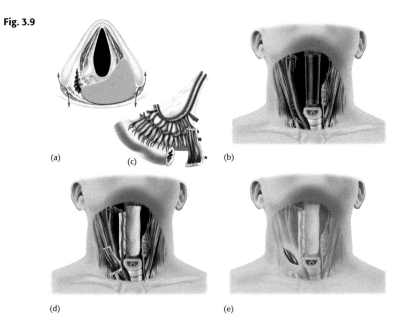

(a)

(c)

(b)

(d)

(e)

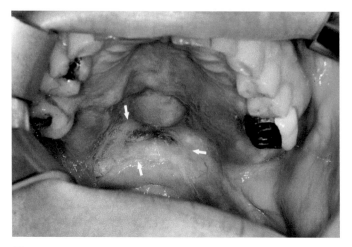

(c)

Fig. 5.16c

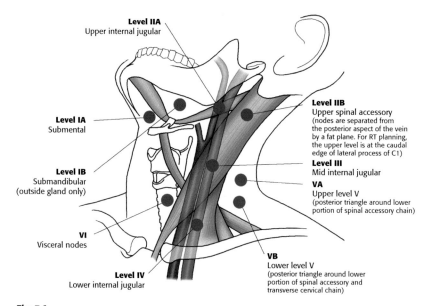

Level IIA
Upper internal jugular

Level IA
Submental

Level IB
Submandibular
(outside gland only)

VI
Visceral nodes

Level IV
Lower internal jugular

Level IIB
Upper spinal accessory
(nodes are separated from
the posterior aspect of the vein
by a fat plane. For RT planning,
the upper level is at the caudal
edge of lateral process of C1)

Level III
Mid internal jugular

VA
Upper level V
(posterior triangle around lower
portion of spinal accessory chain)

VB
Lower level V
(posterior triangle around lower
portion of spinal accessory and
transverse cervical chain)

Fig. 7.1

Fig. 7.2c

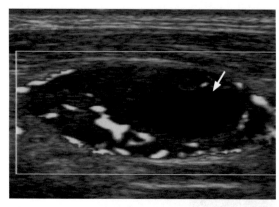

(c)

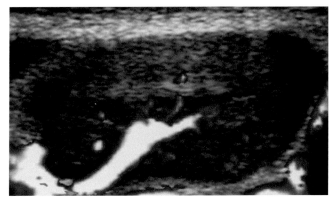

Fig. 7.4a,b

(a)

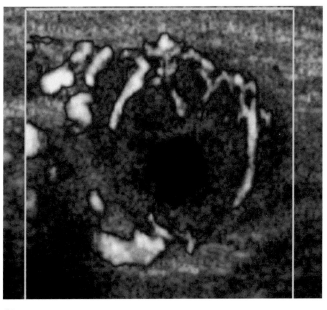

(b)

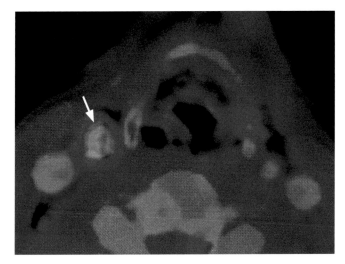

Fig. 7.5a,b

(a)

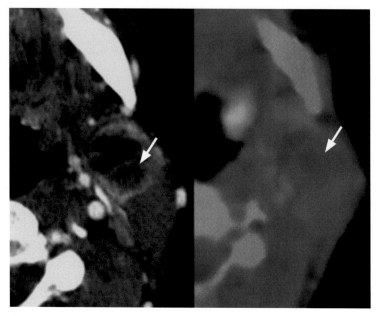

(b)

Fig. 7.5 (cont.)

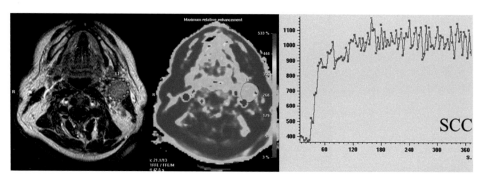

Fig. 7.7

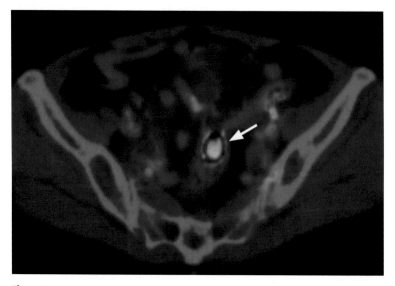

Fig. 7.12

3

Surgery of the orocervical region

Pierre R. Delaere

Introduction

The management of head and neck cancer is a multidisciplinary process. The role of surgery versus radiotherapy and/or chemotherapy in the treatment of head and neck squamous cell cancer largely depends on the localization and stage of the lesion. Imaging findings, essential to determine as precise as possible the local and regional extent of the cancer, may profoundly influence the therapeutic decision process. If surgery is included in the patient management, imaging findings are very helpful in determining the optimal approach and anticipating technical difficulties during resection.

Management of cervical metastasis

The status of the regional lymphatics is one of the most important prognostic indicators in patients with squamous carcinomas arising from the epithelium of the upper aerodigestive tract (oral cavity, oropharynx, hypopharynx and larynx). The presence of regional metastases results in cure rates that are approximately half of those obtainable if metastastes to the regional lymphatic are absent.

In order to establish a consistent and easily reproducible method for description of regional cervical lymph nodes, providing a common language between the clinician, the pathologist and radiologist, the Head and Neck Service at Memorial Sloan-Kettering Cancer Center has described a leveling system for the cervical lymph nodes. This system divides the lymph nodes into seven nodal groups or levels (see also Chs. 1 and 7).

Physical examination of the neck for lymph node metastases has variable reliability [1]. A meta-analysis comparing computed tomography (CT) with physical examination (PE) yielded the following results: sensitivity, 83% (CT) and 74% (PE); specificity, 83% (CT) and 81% (PE); and accuracy, 83% (CT) and 77% (PE). Overall,

Squamous Cell Cancer of the Neck, ed. Robert Hermans. Published by Cambridge University Press.
© R. Hermans 2009.

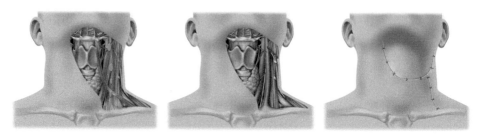

Fig. 3.1. Modified radical neck dissection. The spinal accessory nerve is preserved. Color version in plate section.

PE identified 75% of pathological cervical lymph nodes; this detection rate increased to 91% with addition of CT [2].

The American Joint Committee on Cancer and the International Union against Cancer have agreed upon a uniform staging system for cervical lymph nodes (Chapter 7). An enlarged metastatic cervical lymph node may be the only physical finding present in some patients whose primary tumors are either microscopic or clinically occult at the time of presentation. A systematic search for a primary tumor should be undertaken in these patients prior to embarking upon therapy for the metastatic nodes. If a thorough head and neck examination, including fiberoptic nasolaryngoscopy, CT or magnetic resonance imaging study, and ^{18}F-fluorodeoxyglucose positron emission tomography scan, fail to show a primary tumor, the diagnosis of metastatic carcinoma to a cervical lymph node from an unknown primary is established.

Radical neck dissection, which is defined as the removal of nodal groups I to V with the sternocleidomastoid muscle, internal jugular vein and spinal accessory nerve, is considered to be the standard basic neck dissection. *Modified radical neck dissection* consists of preservation of one or more of the non-lymphatic structures normally removed in the radical procedure (Fig. 3.1). *Selective neck dissection* consists of removal of one or more regional lymph node groups with preservation of the sternocleidomastoid muscle, internal jugular vein and spinal accessory nerve.

Oral cavity cancer

The oral cavity extends posteriorly to the circumvallate papillae of the tongue, the junction of the hard and soft palates, and the anterior faucial arch. The tongue and floor of the mouth are the most common sites of origin for primary squamous cell carcinomas in the oral cavity.

Squamous cell carcinoma may be ulcerative and invasive, fungating and exophytic, or both. The diagnostic evaluation consists of the history and the physical examination, histopathological tissue diagnosis and imaging. Evaluation of the deep extent of the primary tumor and of the neck nodes requires the use of imaging.

The mainstay of treatment of early oral cancer is surgery. Radiation therapy alone can be effective for early superficial lesions but side effects such as xerostomia, as well as potential complications at the level of the mandible, make radiation therapy a poor choice. Usually, surgical resection of the primary tumor is preferred, including a neck dissection to remove the neck nodes at risk.

Advanced T3 and T4 lesions are best treated with a combination of surgery and radiation therapy. Improvement in locoregional control of advanced oral cancer is attributable to the addition of postoperative radiation [3,4].

The defect after resection of small tumors can be closed primarily, healing by secondary intention, or a skin graft can be applied over the defect. Larger defects require a free flap reconstruction to separate the oral cavity from the neck dissection and to preserve a maximal amount of function (Fig. 3.2). The forearm free flap is a fasciocutaneous free flap, based on the radial artery and venae comitantes. It consists of thin, pliable skin and a very long pedicle with large diameter. These characteristics have made it a very useful flap for intraoral and pharyngeal defects [5,6].

Surgical resection of the mandible becomes necessary when a primary malignant tumor of the oral cavity directly extends to the gingiva over the alveolar process, or infiltrates into the mandible. If a primary tumor of the oral cavity approximates the alveolar process, then resection of a part of the mandible ("marginal mandibulectomy"), preserving its arch, is adequate to obtain satisfactory margins around the primary tumor. Mandible reconstruction is not necessary following marginal mandibulectomy.

When resection of an invaded segment of the mandible is indicated, immediate reconstruction of the resected mandible should be considered (Fig. 3.3). The fibula can be transferred as a free osseous or free osseocutaneous flap. The fibula has become the flap of choice for reconstruction of most segmental mandibular defects. The flap is based on the peroneal artery and vein. Because it receives both a segmental and intraosseous blood supply, mutiple osteotomies can be made without devascularizing the bone [7–10].

Tumors of the oropharynx

The oropharynx is that part of the pharynx which extends from the level of the hard palate above to the hyoid bone below. Carcinoma of the oropharynx most

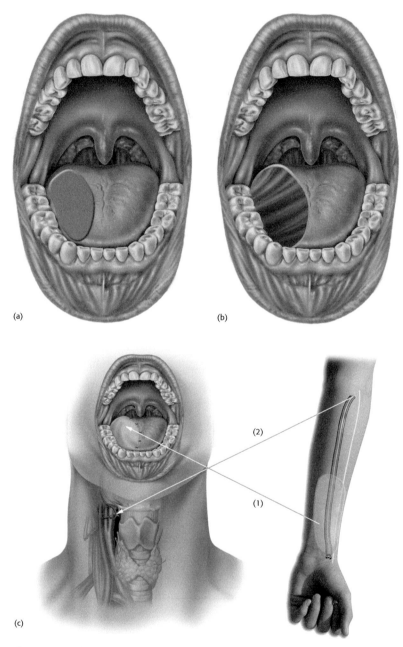

(a)

(b)

(c)

Fig. 3.2. Hemiglossectomy with radial forearm flap reconstruction. (a) The tumor of the oral tongue that requires surgical treatment. (b) The situation after hemiglossectomy. (c) The radial forearm skin (1) is used to reconstruct the hemiglossectomy defect. The radial forearm blood vessels (2) are sutured to the neck vessels to reestablish the blood supply for the radial forearm flap. Color version in plate section.

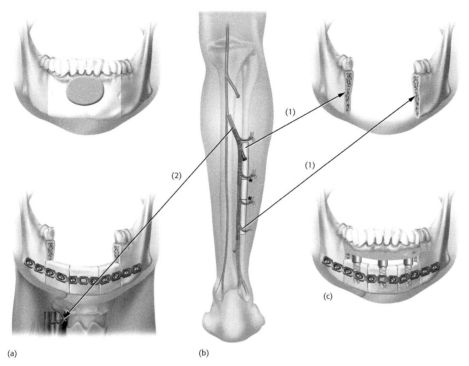

Fig. 3.3. Mandible resection with fibular reconstruction. (a) Schematic presentation of resection of the mandibular symphysis for an extended floor of the mouth tumor with extension into the mandibular bone. (b) Fibular bone is harvested with the peroneal artery and vein. It is osteomized (asterisks) to make the bone into the shape of the mandibular symphysis and placed into the anterior mandibular defect (1); the peroneal blood vessels are sutured to the neck vessels (2). (c) Titanium implants can be placed in the reconstructed mandible to restore the dentition. Color version in plate section.

commonly occurs in the slit between tonsil and base of tongue, at the level of the anterior tonsillar pillar. The initial symptoms of oropharyngeal cancer are often vague and non-specific, leading to a delay in diagnosis. Consequently, the overwhelming majority of patients presents with locally advanced tumors.

Surgery or radiation therapy, alone or in combination, are currently accepted as standard treatment of oropharyngeal cancer. For most patients, the primary treatment consists of (chemo)radiation [11–13].

Surgery is usually reserved for residual or recurrent tumor. The surgical approach must afford good exposure, both for accurate and complete resection of the lesion but also for reconstruction of the defect. Mandibulotomy or mandibular osteotomy is an excellent mandible-sparing surgical approach to gain access to tumors of the oropharynx (Fig. 3.4) [14,15].

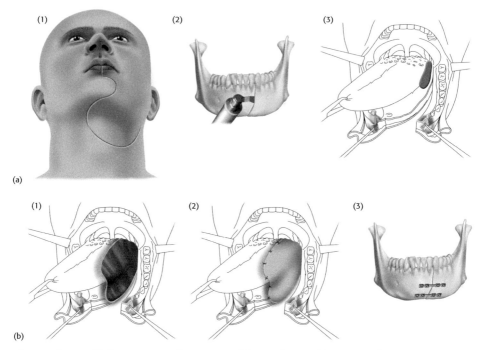

Fig. 3.4. The mandibulotomy approach to tumors of the oropharynx. (a) A paramedian osteotomy (1, 2) can be safely sited between the lateral incisor and the canine teeth to avoid damage or exposure of the dental roots. Incision of the floor of the mouth allows the mandible to be swung out laterally (3) to gain access to the tumor in the oropharynx. (b) Free radial flap reconstruction of the surgical (1, 2) defect after partial resection of the base of the tongue and tonsil. The mandibular osteotomy is fixed using miniplates (3), which provide accurate dental occlusion and stability. Color version in plate section.

The two halves of the mandible are secured in place using miniplates at the end of the procedure.

Patients who have had significant surgical resection and reconstruction require a temporary tracheostomy to protect the airway in the postoperative period.

Tumors of the larynx

The larynx communicates with the oropharynx above and the trachea below. Posteriorly, it is largely surrounded by the hypopharynx. It may be functionally divided into three important areas: supraglottis, glottis and subglottis.

The supraglottis contains the epiglottis, aryepiglottic folds, arytenoids, false cords and includes the laryngeal ventricle. The glottis includes the vocal cords and anterior commissure and posterior commissure.

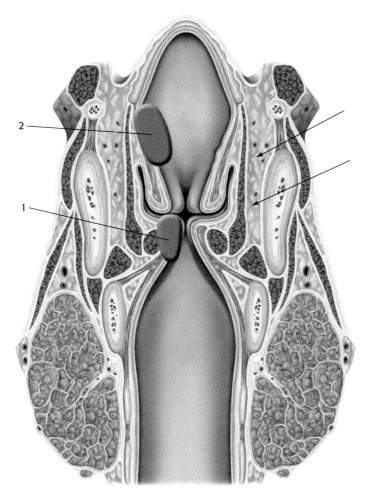

Fig. 3.5. Coronal section of the larynx demonstrating the paraglottic space (arrows). 1, glottic cancer; 2, supraglottic cancer. Color version in plate section.

The most frequent tumor locations are the vocal fold and the supraglottis. Hoarseness is an early symptom of glottic cancer but it may be noticed only later in advanced supraglottic tumors.

The clinical examination of the larynx is limited by the fact that certain areas of the larynx are inaccessible to both visualization and palpation; nevertheless involvement of these structures has an important bearing on staging as well as on management. Information from radiological imaging and operative endoscopy must be utilized in conjunction with physical findings to obtain an accurate pretreatment staging (TNM) record. Supraglottic tumors particularly are frequently understaged because the pre-epiglottic and paraglottic spaces cannot be assessed clinically (Fig. 3.5).

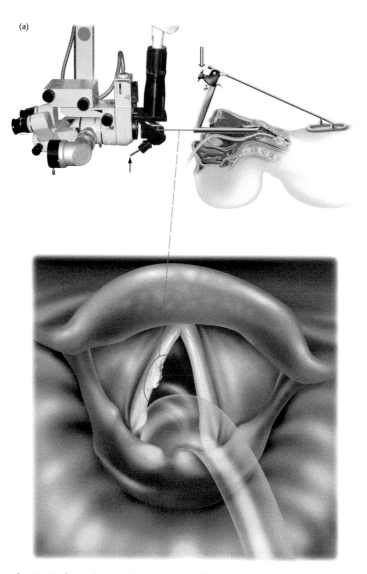

Fig. 3.6. Endoscopic resection of early glottic cancer. (a) Drawing of the intraoperative situation during microlaryngoscopy with a CO_2 laser. The operating microscope is fitted with a micromanipulator (arrow) control of the CO_2 laser beam. The laryngoscope has been introduced transorally and is supported on the platform above the patient's chest. (b) The red line shows extent of laser resection of a T1 glottic cancer. Color version in plate section.

Early lesions can be treated with transoral laser microsurgery (Fig. 3.6) or with radiotherapy, with similar high cure rates [16–18]. The gold standard for advanced lesions (vocal fold fixation) still remains total laryngectomy. Between the proximal trachea and esophagus, a small one-way valve (Provox voice prothesis) is placed,

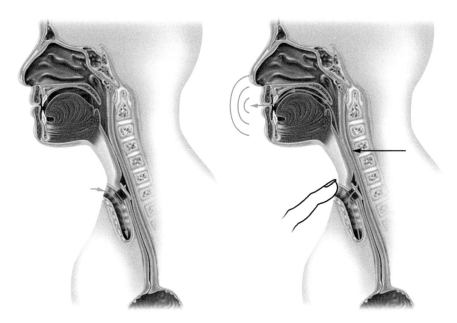

Fig. 3.7. Tracheoesophageal voice after total laryngectomy. (a) Inspiration. (b) Expiration with finger occlusion of the tracheostome. The voice is produced by vibration of the esophageal wall (black arrow). Color version in plate section.

allowing escape of air from the proximal trachea to the esophagus if the tracheostome is closed. In this way the patient has a lot of air available for producing esophageal speech, allowing more rapid speech rehabilitation (Fig. 3.7).

The use of laryngeal preservation schemes with chemoradiotherapy are an important alternative therapy (Chapter 2) [19,20].

If there is clinically apparent lymph node metastasis in the neck and the primary is to be treated by surgery, then a comprehensive neck dissection (levels I to V) should also be performed.

Tumors of the hypopharynx and cervical esophagus

The hypopharynx links the oropharynx superiorly to the larynx and esophagus below. Its boundaries are roughly the hyoid and valleculae above and the cricoid below. Common sites for squamous cell cancers are the pyriform sinuses, the posterior pharyngeal wall and the postcricoid space.

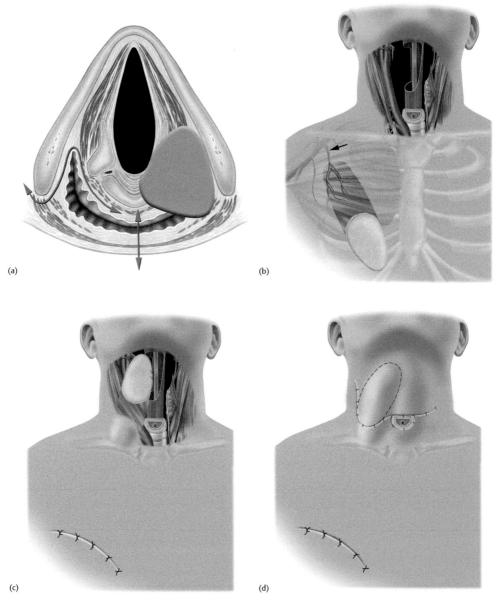

(a)

(b)

(c)

(d)

Fig. 3.8. The pectoralis major flap used for reconstruction of the defect after total laryngectomy with partial pharyngectomy. (a) Schematic representation of laryngopharyngeal tumor with indication of resection margins. (b) Defect after total laryngectomy with partial pharyngectomy. The perfusion sources of the pectoralis major flap are the pectoral branches of the thoracoacromial artery and vein (arrow). (c) Pectoralis flap being sutured into position. (d) Frontal view after reconstruction. Color version in plate section.

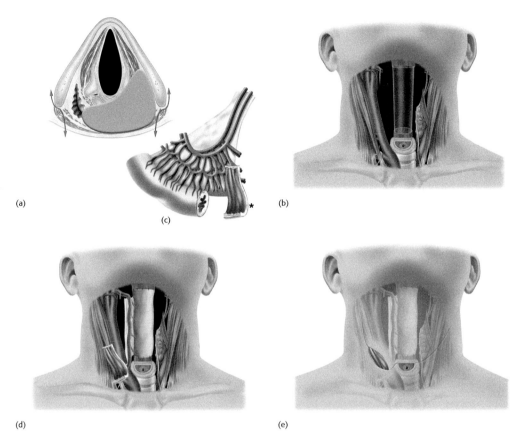

(a)

(b)

(c)

(d)

(e)

Fig. 3.9. Free jejunum transfer after total laryngopharyngectomy. (a) Schematic representation of laryngopharyngeal tumor with indication of resection margins. (b) Frontal view after total laryngopharyngectomy and after placement of a voice prosthesis. A tube reconstuction is necessary to restore the continuity of the alimentary tract. (c) A jejunal tube with a length of 12 cm will be placed in the laryngopharyngectomy defect. A monitor segment (asterisk) is developed by leaving a small segment of jejunum on a mesenteric pedicle. (d) Insetting into the defect is carried out in an isoperistaltic fashion. (e) Situation after transfer of jejunum tube. Color version in plate section.

Treatment options for hypopharyngeal cancer are external radiation therapy, surgery or a combination of these treatment modalities. Currently, an increasing number of patients with hypopharyngeal cancers, otherwise requiring total laryngectomy, are being treated with a larynx preservation treatment program of neoadjuvant or concurrent chemoradiotherapy.

Locally advanced carcinomas of the hypopharynx with extension to the larynx require a wide field total laryngectomy with partial pharyngectomy, as well as a neck dissection.

Partial defects of the hypopharynx can be reconstructed using a pectoralis major myocutaneous flap (Fig. 3.8) [21].

The need for circumferential (total) pharyngectomy depends on the surface extent of the primary tumor. Circumferential defects of the pharynx and cervical esophagus are readily amenable to one-stage reconstruction with a vascularized segment of the intestinal tract (Fig. 3.9) [22].

When the primary tumor extends into the esophagus, the resection includes most or all of the esophagus. For total laryngopharyngo-esophagectomy defects, a gastric pull-up is the reconstruction method of choice [23]. Because of separation of the tracheo-esophageal party wall, speech restoration by placement of a voice prothesis is best carried out as a secondary procedure, ideally a few months after operation.

Conclusions

Management of tumors of the orocervical region has evolved into a complex speciality demanding expertise in various surgical disciplines. In the surgical treatment of this region, there has been increasing emphasis on preservation or restoration of form and function. Function preserving surgical procedures without compromising oncologic effectiveness, as demonstrated in this chapter, are becoming increasingly used.

REFERENCES

1. J. C. Watkinson, D. Johnston, D. Johnston, *et al.* The reliability of palpation in the assessment of tumors. *Clin Otolaryngol* **5** (1990), 405–410.
2. R. M. Merritt, M. F. Williams, T. H. James, E. S. Porubsky. Detection of cervical metastasis. A meta-analysis comparing computed tomography with physical examination. *Arch Otolaryngol Head Neck Surg* **123** (1997), 149–152.
3. B. Vikram, E. W. Strong, P. Shah, R. Spiro. Failure at the primary site following multimodality treatment in advanced head and neck cancer. *Head Neck Surg* **6** (1984), 720–723.
4. B. Vikram, E. W. Strong, J. P. Shah, R. Spiro. Failure in the neck following multimodality treatment in advanced head and neck cancer. *Head Neck Surg* **6** (1984), 724–729.
5. E. Santamaria, F. C. Wei, I. H. Chen, D. C. Chuang. Sensation recovery on innervated radial forearm flap for hemiglossectomy reconstruction by using different recipient nerves. *Plast Reconst Surg* **103** (1999), 450–457.
6. D. S. Soutar, I. A. McGregor. The radial forearm flap in intraoral reconstruction: the experience of 60 consecutive cases. *Plast Reconstr Surg* **78** (1986), 1–8.

7. P. G. Cordeiro, J. J. Disa, D. A. Hidalgo, Q. Y. Hu. Reconstruction of the mandible with osseous free flaps: a ten year experience with 150 consecutive patients. *Plast Reconstr Surg* **104** (1999), 1314–1320.

8. P. G. Cordeiro, D. A. Hidalgo. Conceptual considerations in mandibular reconstruction. *Clin Plast Surg* **22** (1995), 61–69.

9. D. A. Hidalgo. Aesthetic improvements in free-flap mandible reconstruction. *Plast Reconstr Surg* **88** (1991), 574–585.

10. F. C. Wei, C. S. Seah, Y. C. Tsai, S. J. Liu, M. S. Tsai. Fibula osteoseptocutaneous flap for reconstruction of composite mandibular defects. *Plast Reconstr Surg* **93** (1994), 294–304.

11. D. Tong, G. E. Laramore, T. W. Griffen, *et al.* Carcinoma of the tonsil region: results of external irradiation. *Cancer* **49** (1982), 2009–2014.

12. D. A. Fein, R. W. Lee, W. R. Amos, *et al.* Oropharyngeal carcinoma treated with radiotherapy: a 30-year experience. *Int J Radiat Oncol Biol Phys* **34** (1996), 289–296.

13. J. T. Parsons, W. M. Mendenhall, R. R. Million, S. P. Stringer. The management of primary cancers of the oropharynx: combined treatment or irradiation alone? *Semin Radiat Oncol* **2** (1992), 142–148.

14. R. H. Spiro, F. P. Gerold, J. P. Shah, R. B. Sessions, E. W. Strong. Mandibulotomy approach to oropharyngeal tumors. *Am J Surg*, **150** (1985), 466–469.

15. R. H. Spiro, F. P. Gerold, E. W. Strong. Mandibular "swing" approach for oral and oropharyngeal tumors. *Head Neck Surg* **3** (1981), 371–378.

16. C. Sittel, H. E. Eckel, C. Eschenburg. Phonatory results after laser surgery for glottic carcinoma. *Otolaryngol Head Neck Surg* **119** (1998), 419–424.

17. E. N. Myers, R. L. Wagner, J. T. Johnson. Microlaryngoscopic surgery for T1 glottic lesions: a cost-effective option. *Ann Otol Rhinol Laryngol* **103** (1994), 28–30.

18. D. A. Fein, W. M. Mendenhall, J. T. Parsons, R. R. Million. T_1T_2 squamous cell carcinoma of the glottic larynx treated with radiotherapy: a multivariate analysis of variables potentially influencing local control. *Int J Radiat Oncol Biol Phys* **25** (1993), 605–611.

19. S. G. Urba, A. A. Forastiere, G. T. Wolf, *et al.* Intensive induction chemotherapy and radiation for organ preservation in patients with advanced resectable head and neck carcinoma. *J Clin Oncol* **12** (1994), 946–953.

20. W. M. Mendenhall, J. T. Parsons, S. P. Stringer, N. J. Cassisi, R. R. Million. Stage T_3 squamous cell carcinoma of the glottic larynx: a comparison of laryngectomy and irradiation. *Int J Radiat Oncol Biol Phys* **23** (1992), 725–732.

21. R. Fabian. Pectoralis major myocutaneous flap reconstruction of the laryngopharynx and cervical esophagus. *Laryngoscope* **98** (1988), 1227–1231.

22. D. R. Thiele, D. W. Robinson, D. E. Thiele, W. B. Coman. Free jejunal interposition reconstruction after pharyngolaryngectomy: 201 consecutive cases. *Head Neck* **83** (1995), 83–88.

23. C. E. Cahow, C. T. Sasaki. Gastric pull-up reconstruction for pharyngo-laryngo-esophagectomy. *Arch Surg* **129** (1994), 425–429.

4

Laryngeal and hypopharyngeal cancer

Frédérique Dubrulle, Raphaëlle Souillard, Dominique Chevalier and
Philippe Puech

Introduction

Laryngeal and hypopharyngeal neoplasms are squamous cell carcinomas in up to
95% of patients. The most important established risk factor is chronic use of tobacco
and alcohol, especially when used in combination. The evaluation of laryngeal and
hypopharyngeal tumor extension is based on clinical examination, endoscopic examination and computed tomographic (CT) imaging. Spiral CT and, more recently,
multidetector CT offer an accurate examination of the upper aerodigestive tract with
the advantage of rapid acquisition of data in a highly reproducible way.

Computed tomographic technique

Scan issues

The primary role of imaging is to evaluate local and locoregional tumor extension,
in conjunction with the clinical examination [1,2]. It is important to evaluate the
entire aerodigestive tract because multiple sites of tumor are not rare in these
patients. Consequently, CT images are acquired from the nasopharynx to the
cervicomediastinal junction.Using multidetector CT (MDCT), images can then be
reconstructed to approximately 1 mm. Multiplanar reformatting is then possible for
the pharyngolaryngeal area and the cervical lymph nodes areas [3,4].

The CT study can be extended to include the thoracomediastinal area to look for
other primary tumors or metastatic lesions.

The advantages of modern MDCT include [1,3]:

exploration of the entire pharyngolaryngeal area in a short acquisition time (< 20 s)

reduction of motion and deglutition artefacts

the possibility of obtaining images during phonation or the Valsalva maneuver

the ability to perform multiplanar reformatting in the coronal or sagittal planes

Squamous Cell Cancer of the Neck, ed. Robert Hermans. Published by Cambridge University Press.
© R. Hermans 2009.

optimization of scan timing to obtain optimal tissue contrast medium, particularly relating to the neck vessels
comprehensive evaluation of the neck lymph nodes, from the skull base to the supraclavicular area.

Scan protocol and practical modalities

It is recommended that the CT study is performed before biopsy, particularly for small tumors as the resultant inflammatory reaction may obscure the tumor. The CT study should be acquired either before a direct laryngoscopic examination or about 10 to 15 days after biopsy in case of a small tumor.

The first acquisition (over about 15 cm) should extend from the nasopharynx down to the first centimeters of the cervical trachea. The raw data are reformatted and reconstructed in a stack of thin and overlapping images. For this first acquisition, the images are obtained during quiet respiration. Breath-holding is not recommended because it induces closing of the glottis, resulting in less optimal evaluation of the vocal cords. The patient is asked not to swallow as this will avoid motion artefacts. In our institution, this first acquisition is acquired after intravenous injection of 80 ml of contrast agent. The injection is biphasic: 50 ml at 1 ml/s, then with 30 s between the two phases, 30 ml at 2 ml/s. The acquisition begins just after the second bolus injection. This technique provides optimal tissue enhancement, allowing correct discrimination between tumoral and normal tissue, and good definition of the neck vessels [3].

Laryngeal and hypopharyngeal tumors usually appear as an enhancing, infiltrating or exophytic mass, sometimes ulcerated, creating an asymmetry of the laryngeal soft tissues [2].

Dynamic maneuvers

Dynamic maneuvers can provide important additional information and are performed separately from the routine scans described above during a second acquisition. We choose the most appropriate maneuver adapted to the pathology: the phonation maneuver is preferred for laryngeal tumors, while the Valsalva maneuver is used for hypopharyngeal tumors.

Phonation
The patient is asked to produce a high-pitched "eeee" sound. This maneuver is used for analysis of laryngeal mobility and for better visualization of the aryepiglottic

Table 4.1. Subsites within the larynx

Regions	Subsites
Supraglottis	Suprahyoid epiglottis (including tip, lingual and laryngeal surfaces)
	Infrahyoid epiglottis
	Aryepiglottic fold, laryngeal aspect
	Arytenoid
	Ventricular bands (false vocal cords)
Glottis	True vocal cords
	Anterior commissure
	Posterior commissure
Subglottis	

From Sobin and Wittekind, 2002 [5].

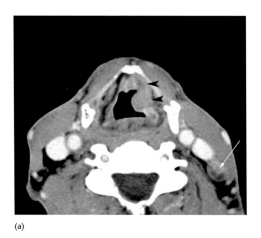
(a)

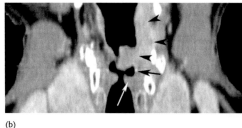
(b)

Fig. 4.1. Patient presenting with a left supraglottic tumor. (a) The tumor extends to the false vocal cord and deep into the paralaryngeal space (arrowhead). Note the presence of a left midjugular (level III) adenopathy (arrow). (b) Coronal reconstruction during phonation shows no extension to the glottic level (white arrow) and correct opening of the laryngeal ventricle (arrow). The tumor (arrowheads) is limited to the supraglottic level.

folds. During phonation, the laryngeal ventricles open, allowing clearer subdivision of the larynx in its three anatomical regions: supraglottic, glottic and subglottic (Table 4.1). These three areas are well delineated on coronal reconstructions (Figs. 4.1 and 4.2). This subdivision of the larynx into three levels is useful for staging of a laryngeal tumor, as a tumor extending to another level is classified as T2 in the International Union against Cancer (UICC) 2002 classification (Tables 4.2 and 4.3) [5].

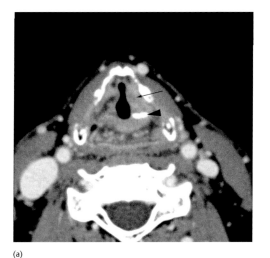

(a)

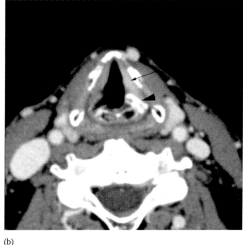

(b)

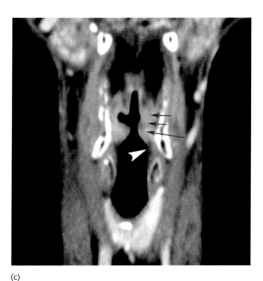

(c)

Fig. 4.2. Extension of a supraglottic tumor to the glottic level. (a) Patient presenting with a left false vocal cord tumor (arrow) with sclerosis of the left arytenoid cartilage (arrowhead). (b) Enhancement of the left true vocal cord (arrow) with sclerosis of the homolateral arytenoid cartilage (arrowhead). (c) Coronal reconstruction during phonation shows the extension of this supraglottic tumor (upper short arrow) to the left laryngeal ventricle, which does not expand (lower short arrow), and enhancement of the left true vocal cord (long arrow). The subglottis is not affected by tumor (white arrowhead).

This subdivision of the larynx is also useful to understand the different laryngeal surgical techniques, especially partial horizontal laryngectomies.

Valsalva maneuver

The Valsalva maneuver is systematically used for the study of the hypopharynx [3,4] and involves the closing of the glottis and hypopharyngeal distension, leading to dilatation of the piriform sinuses and better visualization of the aryepiglottic folds. The distension induced by this maneuver may extend into the retrocricoarytenoid region.

Table 4.2. Tumor staging of laryngeal carcinomas in the International Union Against Cancer 2002 classification

Stage	Description
T1	
T1 supraglottic	Tumor limited to one subsite of the supraglottis with normal vocal cord mobility
T1 glottic	Tumor limited to vocal cord(s) with normal mobility (may involve anterior and posterior commissure)
T1a	Tumor limited to one vocal cord
T1b	Tumor involving both vocal cords
T1 subglottic	Tumor limited to the subglottis with normal vocal cord mobility
T2	
T2 supraglottic	Tumor invading mucosa of more than one adjacent subsite of supraglottis, glottis or extraglottic region (base of tongue mucosa, vallecula, medial face of piriform sinus)
T2 glottic	Glottic tumor with extension to subglottis or supraglottis and/or with impaired vocal cord mobility (without laryngeal fixation)
T2 subglottic	Subglottic tumor extending to vocal cords with normal or impaired vocal cord mobility
T3	Tumor limited to laryngeal area with vocal cord fixation and/or invasion of the retrocricoid area, and/or the pre-epiglottic space, and/or the paraglottic space, and/or minor erosion of internal perichondrium of thyroid cartilage
T4	Cartilage extension and/or extralaryngeal tumor spread
T4a	Tumor invading thyroid cartilage and/or extralaryngeal structures: trachea, soft tissues of the neck (including deep muscles of the tongue: genioglossus muscle, hyoglossus muscle, palatoglossus muscle and styloglossus muscle), subhyoid muscles, thyroid gland, esophagus
T4b	Tumor invading prevertebral space, mediastinal structures or encasing carotid artery

From Sobin and Wittekind, 2002 [5].

In our experience, it is important that the patient practises any maneuver before the actual CT examination, as this will increase the likelihood of its success.

During such a dynamic maneuver, the acquisition is focused on the pharyngo-laryngeal area, with a shorter acquisition time (less than 10 s with MDCT), and the biphasic injection of 80 ml of contrast agent is repeated before this acquisition [3].

We systematically perform a chest CT to look for other primary tumors such as lung or esophageal, lung metastasis or mediastinal metastatic lymph node

Table 4.3. Tumor staging of hypopharyngeal carcinomas in the International Union Against Cancer 2002 classification

Stage	Description
T1	Tumor limited to one hypopharyngeal subsite and 2 cm or less in greatest dimension
T2	Tumor invading more than one subsite of the hypopharynx and/or an adjacent site (aryepiglottic fold, posterior pharyngeal wall, retrocricoarytenoid area), and/or > 2 cm but < 4 cm in greatest dimension without fixation of the hemilarynx
T3	Tumor with fixation of the hemilarynx and/or measuring > 4 cm in greatest dimension
T4	Tumor invades thyroid/cricoid cartilage, hyoid bone, thyroid gland, esophagus or central compartment soft tissues

From Sobin and Wittekind, 2002 [5].

infiltration. In our experience, if thoracic abnormalities are detected on the chest CT study, such findings lead to a management change in 10% of patients.

Laryngeal carcinomas

Supraglottic carcinomas

Supraglottic carcinomas occur at four main sites: the laryngeal surface of the epiglottis, the laryngeal aditus, the false cords (also called ventricular bands) and Morgagni's ventricle (also called laryngeal ventricle).

Possible extension to the glottic level must be carefully sought especially when partial horizontal laryngectomy, such as cricohyoidoepiglottopexy (CHEP) or crico-hyoidopexy (CHP), is being considered. For optimal differentiation of the glottic from the supraglottic level, CT must be performed during phonation, causing opening of the laryngeal ventricles. This distinction is particularly well documented on coronal reconstructions (Figs. 4.1 and 4.2). Surgical management of a purely supraglottic tumor differs from that for a supraglottic tumor extending to the glottic level [6].

Tumoral extension superiorly to the valleculae and the base of tongue is important to detect, especially in tumors of the free margin of the epiglottis. Optimal tissue enhancement and sagittal reconstructions through the base of tongue are important for this evaluation. If extension is present, it is important to evaluate how deep it is, especially when partial resection of the base of tongue is being considered (Fig. 4.3).

One of the primary roles of imaging in patients with supraglottic tumor is to provide information on submucosal extension of the primary tumor, especially to

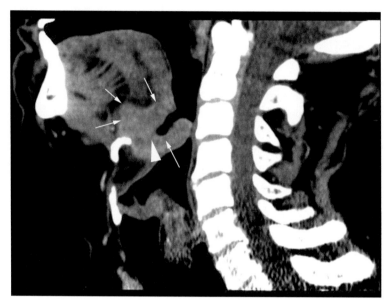

Fig. 4.3. Sagittal reconstruction illustrating a tumor of the free margin of the epiglottis with extension to the vallecula (arrowhead) and to the base of the tongue (arrows).

the pre-epiglottic space, which cannot be evaluated clinically [7,8]. A CT scan is used to detect such submucosal extension in the pre-epiglottic space in tumors of the laryngeal surface of the epiglottis, tumors at the base of the epiglottis and tumors of the false vocal cords [6,9]. Infiltration of the pre-epiglottic space is well demonstrated on axial images and also on sagittal reconstructions, and the degree of infiltration, from limited to total, must be specified (Figs. 4.4 and 4.5).

Computer tomography is also performed to evaluate laryngeal cartilage invasion. Cartilage abnormalities are less commonly seen in supraglottic cancers than in glottic cancers. Three features of cartilage involvement can be seen on CT [10,11,12].

Sclerosis is frequently observed (Figs. 4.2; also 4.7 and 4.9, below). When sclerosis is present, it correlates with invasion of the arytenoid in 25% of patients and invasion of the cricoid cartilage in 50% of cases [1,11]. So this sign alone is not specific for cartilage invasion, often indicating reactive bone formation as a result of the tumor in contact with the cartilage.

Erosion is a specific criterion for tumoral invasion and indicates a T3 tumor. It can be seen well on reconstructions using a "cartilage" window/center setting (1400–400 UH) (Fig. 4.8, below). Cartilage erosion is sometimes difficult to evaluate because of a large variability in the ossification pattern of the laryngeal cartilages, especially the thyroid cartilage [11].

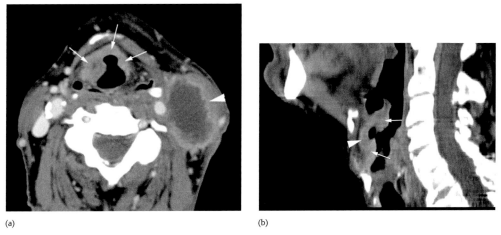

(a)   (b)

Fig. 4.4. Patient presenting with an ulcerated tumor of the laryngeal face of the epiglottis. (a) The tumor is indicated with arrows. There is a midjugular left necrotic lymph node (arrowhead) with thrombosis of the jugular vein and close contact with the carotid artery. (b) Sagittal reconstruction shows tumoral extension into the pre-epiglottic space (arrowhead).

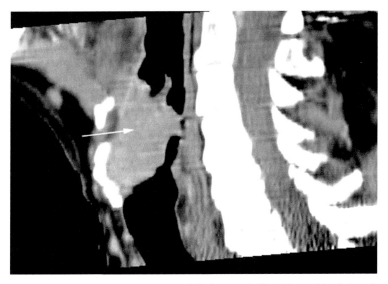

Fig. 4.5. Massive extension of a tumor of the laryngeal side of the epiglottis into the entire pre-epiglottic space (arrow).

Lysis, a sign of major cartilage invasion (Fig. 4.9, below), is well detected on CT scan, even without using a "cartilage" window. The tumor is considered as T4 tumor in such cases. The presence of a tumor on the extralaryngeal side of the cartilage has to be evaluated in these circumstances (Fig. 4.9, below).

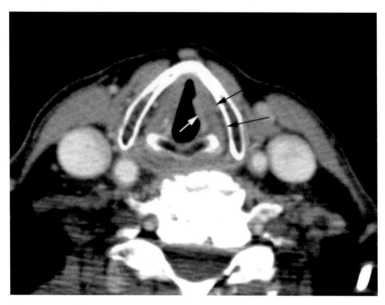

Fig. 4.6. Superficial tumor of the posterior two thirds of the left true vocal cord (white arrow) without deep extension to the paraglottic space (black arrows).

Glottic carcinomas

In glottic carcinoma, it is important to evaluate the anteroposterior extension (Fig. 4.6), particularly whether or not it extends into the anterior commissure (Figs. 4.7 and 4.8), which appears as tissue thickening at this level, in contact with the thyroid cartilage. If the tumor has extended to the anterior commissure, further extension is possible to the controlateral true vocal cord, the thyroid cartilage, the base of the epiglottis and the pre-epiglottic space (Fig. 4.8). Possible extension to the posterior commissure has also to be identified. Extension to the anterior or posterior commissure is analyzed on images acquired during quiet respiration.

It is important to evaluate the possibility of deep extension, as this largely determines the staging of the tumor and the most appropriate treatment [13]. Extension to the vocal muscle and obliteration of the paraglottic fat, adjacent to the thyroid cartilage, is seen in infiltrative tumors (Fig. 4.7); sclerosis of the thyroid cartilage is a good sign for tumoral contact with the cartilage.

Extension to the pre-epiglottic space has also to be sought; such an extension indicates a T3 tumor [7,13].

As with supraglottic tumors, laryngeal cartilage invasion has to be identified and the CT features are the same as those described above (Fig. 4.8). Extension to the cartilage

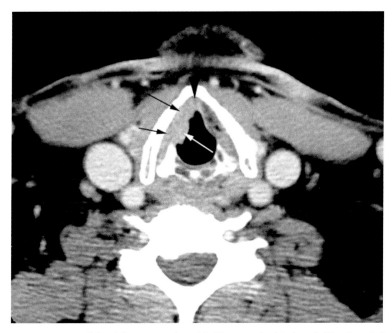

Fig. 4.7. Tumor of the right true vocal cord (white arrow) with deep infiltration of the paraglottic space (black arrows) and extension in the anterior commissure (arrowhead). Note the sclerosis of the right arytenoid cartilage.

corresponds to a T4 tumor, except for erosions limited to the internal perichondrium (T3) (Table 4.2) [5]. Several studies have shown that radiotherapy or chemoradiotherapy is less successful in tumors with clear cartilage invasion [14,15].

Extralaryngeal extension through lytic cartilage indicates a T4 tumor. In glottic tumors, prelaryngeal extension is regarded as an indication for total laryngectomy, including resection of the prelaryngeal tissues (Fig. 4.9).

Tumoral extension deep to the mucosa is well depicted on imaging, whereas it is difficult to detect with laryngoscopy [13], except in cases of vocal cord immobility, which is an indirect sign of deep tumor extension. Deep tumor extension has to be identified on imaging because of staging and management consequences.

Coronal reconstructions from images acquired during phonation are helpful to demonstrate cephalad extension to the laryngeal ventricle and the false vocal cord. Subglottic extension of a glottic carcinoma often contraindicates partial laryngectomy [2,16]. This appears as contrast-enhanced thickening in continuity with the glottic tumor, close to the cricoid cartilage. Sclerosis of the cricoid cartilage indicates the presence of tumor close to the cartilage. Coronal reconstructions allow precise measurement of subglottic extension (Fig. 4.10).

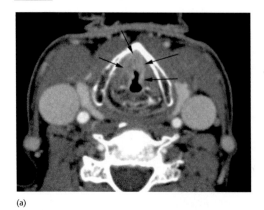 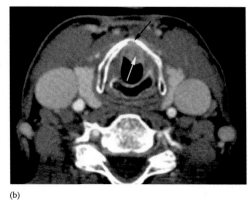

(a)   (b)

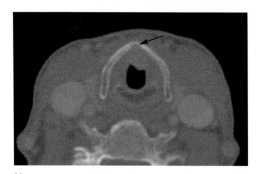

(c)

Fig. 4.8. Tumor affecting the three levels of the larynx. (a) Infiltrative tumor of the right true vocal cord, extending to the anterior commissure and the controlateral true vocal cord (black arrows). (b) Axial CT image obtained at lower level shows anterior subglottic extension (white arrow) with erosion of the thyroid cartilage (black arrow). (c) Erosion of the thyroid cartilage is best depicted on an image with "cartilage" window.

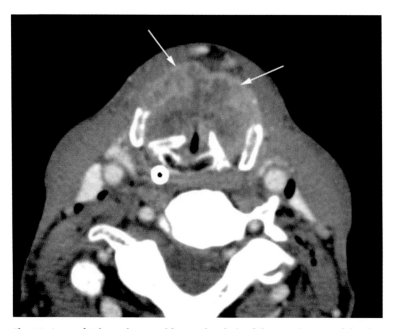

Fig. 4.9. Large glottic carcinoma with complete lysis of the anterior part of the thyroid cartilage and tumoral extension into the prelaryngeal tissues (arrows).

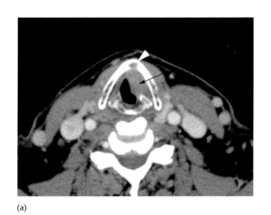

(a)

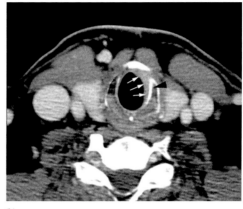

(b)

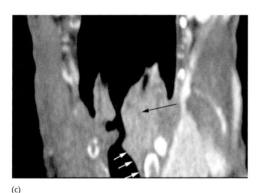

(c)

Fig. 4.10. **(a) Infiltrative tumor of the left true vocal cord (black arrow), causing lysis of the thyroid cartilage in contact with the anterior commissure (white arrowhead). (b) Subglottic extension (white arrows) with sclerosis of the adjacent cricoid cartilage (black arrowhead). (c) Coronal reconstruction acquired during phonation shows the importance of the subglottic extension (white arrows). Note also the supraglottic extension (black arrow).**

Subglottic carcinomas

Primary subglottic tumors are rare. Cancer at the level of the subglottis often corresponds to subglottic extension of a glottic tumor.

Primary tumors of the subglottis are often infiltrative, presenting with invasion of the cricoid cartilage and/or extralaryngeal extension, possibly involving adjacent soft tissues such as the thyroid gland. Tracheal involvement has to be ruled out.

Hypopharyngeal carcinomas

Superficial tumoral extension

Malignant hypopharyngeal tumors are squamous cell carcinomas in up to 95% of patients.

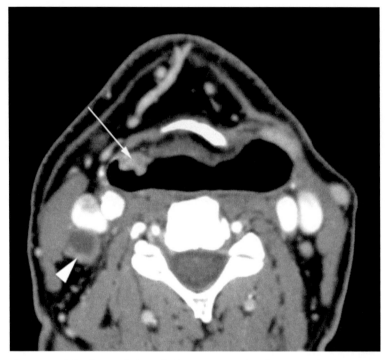

Fig. 4.11. Axial CT image during Valsalva maneuver, showing an exophytic tumor (arrow) of the anterior wall of the right piriform sinus. Note the presence of a centrally necrotic adenopathy on the right (arrowhead).

The role of imaging is for accurate tumoral mapping and detection of possible extension on which to plan appropriate treatment [2,10].

The hypopharynx is divided into three regions: the piriform sinuses, the posterior pharyngeal wall and the retrocricoarytenoid area. The hypopharynx is in continuity with the esophagus. Piriform sinus tumors are the most frequent hypopharyngeal carcinomas.

The Valsalva maneuver, inducing the opening of the piriform sinuses, may allow an easier visualization of superficial extension to the anterior, lateral and posterior walls of the piriform sinus (Figs. 4.11 and 4.12). Extension to the posterior pharyngeal wall has to be carefully sought, especially to the midline (Fig. 4.12).

Superior extension to the oropharynx, including the base of the tongue, may be present.

Extension to the retrocricoarytenoid area has to be searched for (Figs. 4.13 and 4.14). The inferior limit of the hypopharynx is located at the level of the inferior part of the cricoid cartilage. At this level the hypopharynx loses its ovoid shape, merging

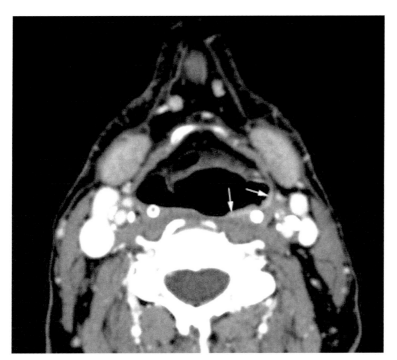

Fig. 4.12. Axial CT image acquired during Valsalva maneuver, showing a superficial tumor of the posterolateral wall of the left piriform sinus (arrows). The tumor almost crosses the midline at the level of the posterior pharyngeal wall.

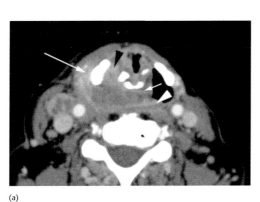

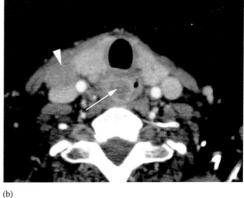

(a)   (b)

Fig. 4.13. A patient with a large tumor of the right piriform sinus. (a) There is extension to the retrocricoarytenoid area (short white arrow), extending over the midline at the level of the posterior pharyngeal wall (white arrowhead). Note the endolaryngeal extension (black arrow head) and the extralaryngeal extension along the inferior constrictor pharyngeal muscle (long white arrow). (b) Submucosal extension to the cervical esophagus (arrow). Note the right low jugular lymphadenopathy (arrowhead).

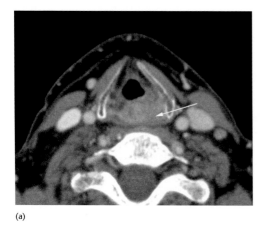 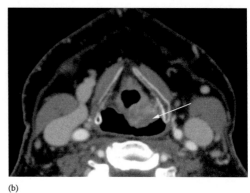

(a)   (b)

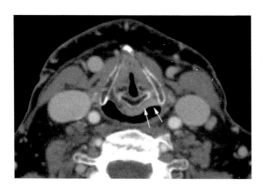

(c)

Fig. 4.14. Hypopharyngeal tumor. (a) The tumor is evident in the lower part of the hypopharynx (arrow). (b) Axial CT acquired during Valsalva maneuver shows that the tumor arises from the anterior wall of the piriform sinus (arrow). (c) Extension to the retrocricoarytenoid area (arrows) can be seen.

with the round- to oval-shaped esophagus. It is important to look for evidence of extension to the cervical esophagus, as evidenced by abnormal enhancement and/or soft tissue thickening (Fig. 4.13). Extension to the cervical esophagus influences the therapeutic options: total pharyngolaryngectomy is not possible and partial resection of the esophagus with gastric pull-up has to be performed.

Deep tumoral extension

The primary role of imaging in head and neck cancers is to evaluate deep mucosal extension. Anteriorly, a piriform sinus tumor often extends into the larynx [3,10], especially to the posterior part of the paraglottic space; this results in widening of the thyroarytenoid gap and infiltration of the posterior part of the true and/or the false vocal cord (Figs. 4.13 and 4.15). Infiltration of the pre-epiglottic space can be seen in advanced

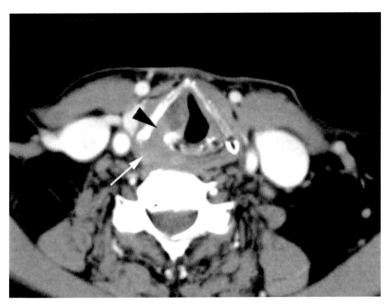

Fig. 4.15. Tumor of the lower part of the right piriform sinus (white arrow) with intralaryngeal extension to the posterior part of the right true vocal cord. Note the widening of the thyroarytenoid gap (arrowhead) and the sclerosis of the adjacent cartilages.

tumors. Deep extension to the prevertebral fascia and muscles must be sought, with particular attention paid for tumors of the posterior pharyngeal wall (Fig. 4.16).

As elsewhere, cartilaginous extension [2,10] is important to detect in hypopharyngeal tumors, especially in tumors of the lateral or anterior wall of the piriform sinus. The tumor may reach the thyroid ala, eventually causing its destruction. The criteria for neoplastic involvement of the cartilages are as described above.

From the piriform sinus, the tumor may extend beyond the pharyngeal structures, most often along the inferior pharyngeal constrictor muscle (whose fibers attach along the lateral surface of the thyroid cartilage wing, Fig. 4.13), invading the soft tissues of the neck; the carotid artery is at risk of becoming involved. Optimal tumor and vessel enhancement allows correct evaluation of such extralaryngeal/extrapharyngeal extension. Direct extralaryngeal extension through an area of cartilage lysis is less common.

Lymphatic extension

Neck nodal metastasis is very common in pharyngolaryngeal carcinomas, especially supraglottic carcinomas and hypopharyngeal carcinomas [4,17].

The imaging criteria for diagnosing nodal metastases are discussed in Ch. 7.

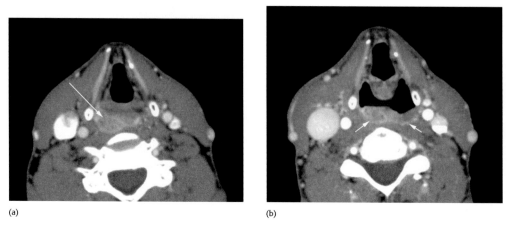

(a)   (b)

Fig. 4.16. Axial CT images. (a) Image acquired during quiet breathing shows tumoral enhancement of the hypopharynx (arrow). (b) The image during Valsalva maneuver shows that the tumor is localized in the pharyngeal posterior wall; involvement of the prevertebral fascia cannot be excluded (arrows).

Many studies have shown no significant difference between magnetic resonance imaging (MRI) and CT in detecting cervical metastatic lymph nodes [18,19]. Most authors suggest using the same technique as used for primary tumor evaluation to analyze the neck lymph nodes. The CT scan is the recommended technique for laryngeal and hypopharyngeal carcinomas [19]. One of the major advantages of CT is that a complete study of all lymphatic areas, from the skull base to the mediastinum, is possible. The presence of retropharyngeal adenopathies modifies the therapeutic management.

Metastatic nodes from hypopharyngeal carcinomas are often of large diameter and present with capsular penetration. The role of imaging is to search for contraindications regarding their surgical resection. Therefore, the relationship of the tumor to the carotid artery must be studied carefully (the jugular vein, thrombosed in most cases, is removed during surgery). Optimal opacification of the vessels allows differentiation and better analysis of the relationship between the lymphadenopathy and the carotid artery. It is necessary to specify the contact surface, the presence or not of a fatty space between them and the degree to which the tumor encircles the artery [17].

Magnetic resonance imaging

The use of MRI is very helpful for the evaluation of many head and neck tumors, but not for laryngeal and hypopharyngeal carcinomas. The main disadvantages of MRI, when compared with MDCT, are the long acquisition time (a source of motion artefacts), less-optimal spatial resolution and the limited anatomical region covered (whereas the entire upper aerodigestive tract is imaged in a single CT study).

There are a few specific circumstances where MRI is useful: MRI of the larynx is the best method to detect neoplastic cartilage invasion or deep tumoral extension to the true vocal cord [8,16] and MRI is a more sensitive technique than CT for detection of cartilage abnormalities [14,15,20,21]. When laryngeal conservation therapy is considered, MRI may be helpful to exclude cartilaginous involvement.

Cartilaginous invasion shows high signal intensity on T_2-weighted images and enhancement on contrast-enhanced T_1-weighted images. However, these signal changes are not specific and may also be seen in peritumoral inflammation. Because of this, MRI gives more false-positive results than CT [15,21].

In the new UICC classification for laryngeal tumors, modified in 2002 [5], a laryngeal tumor with limited cartilaginous invasion is considered a T3 tumor instead of T4, which does not contraindicate conservative treatment for those tumors. Large cartilage lysis is easily detected on CT and corresponds to a T4 tumor; a tumor associated with limited cartilage erosion on CT will be classified as a T3 tumor. Therefore, taking into consideration this modified classification of laryngeal tumors, the indications to perform a MRI study are not common.

Conclusions

Nowadays, the radiological evaluation of laryngeal and hypopharyngeal cancer is achieved with multidetector CT, which offers a complete locoregional tumor evaluation and can include imaging of the thorax, a common area of metastatic disease or second primary tumors. To obtain high-quality imaging studies, sufficient attention has to be given to technical factors, including information to the patient and precise timing of the contrast agent injection.

REFERENCES

1. F. Dubrulle, Y. Robert, C. Delerue. Intérêt du scanner spiralé dans la pathologie du larynx et de l'hypopharynx. *Feuill radiolog* **37** (1997), 118–131.
2. R. Hermans. Staging of laryngeal and hypopharyngeal cancer: value of imaging studies. *Eur Radiol* **16** (2006), 2386–2400.
3. F. Dubrulle, D. Chevalier. Imagerie par scanner hélicoïdal des cancers de l'hypopharynx. Les cahiers d'ORL. T. XXXVI n° 1 (2003).

4. D. Chevalier, F. Dubrulle, B. Vilette. Anatomie descriptive, endoscopique et radiologique du larynx. In *Encyclopédie Médico Chirurgicale* (Paris: Elsevier, 20-630-A-10 2001).

5. L. H. Sobin, C. Wittekind (eds.) *UICC TNM Classification of Malignant Tumors*, 6th edn (New York: Wiley-Liss, 2002), p. 36.

6. A. A. Mancuso, S. K. Mukherji, I. Chmalfuss, *et al.* Preradiotherapy computed tomography as a predictor of local control in supraglottic carcinoma. *J Clin Oncol* **17** (1999), 631–637.

7. M. Becker. Larynx and hypopharynx. *Radiol Clin North Am* **36** (1998), 891–920.

8. P. D. Phelps. Review: carcinoma of the larynx. The role of imaging in staging and pre treatment. *Clin Radiol* **46** (1993), 77–83.

9. D. E. Freeman, A. A. Mancuso, J. T. Parsons, W. M. Mendenhall, R. R. Million. Irradiation alone for supraglottic larynx carcinoma: can CT findings predict treatment results? *Int J Radiat Oncol Biol Phys* **19** (1990), 485–490.

10. P. Zbären, M. Becker, H. Lang. Pretherapeutic staging of hypopharyngeal carcinoma. Clinical findings, computed tomography, and magnetic resonance imaging compared with histopathologic evaluation. *Arch Otolaryngol Head Neck Surg* **123** (1997), 908–913.

11. M. Becker, P. Zbären, J. Delavelle, *et al.* Neoplastic invasion of the laryngeal cartilage: reassessment of criteria for diagnosis at CT. *Radiology* **203** (1997), 521–532.

12. H. D. Curtin. Importance of imaging demonstration of neoplastic invasion of laryngeal cartilage. *Radiology* **194** (1995), 643–644.

13. S. K. Mukherji, A. A. Mancuso, W. Mendenhall, *et al.* Can pretreatment CT predict local control of T$_2$ glottic carcinomas treated with radiation therapy alone? *Am J Neuroradiol* **16** (1995), 655–662.

14. M. Becker. Neoplastic invasion of laryngeal cartilage: radiologic diagnosis and therapeutic implications. *Eur J Radiol* **33** (2000), 216–229.

15. J. A. Castelijns, M. Becker, R. Hermans. Impact of cartilage invasion on treatment and prognosis of laryngeal cancer. *Eur Radiol* **6** (1996), 156–169.

16. R. Hermans. Laryngeal neoplasms. In *Head and Neck Cancer Imaging*, ed. R. Hermans (Berlin: Springer, 2006), pp. 43–80.

17. L. Barbera, P. A. Groome, W. J. Mackillop, *et al.* The role of computed tomography in the T classification of laryngeal carcinoma. *Cancer* **91** (2001), 394–407.

18. H. J. Steinkamp, N. Hosten, C. Richter, *et al.* Enlarged cervical lymph nodes at helical CT. *Radiology* **191** (1994), 795–798.

19. J. Castelijns, M. van den Brekel. Neck nodal disease. In *Head and Neck Cancer Imaging*, ed. R. Hermans (Berlin: Springer, 2006), pp. 293–310.

20. H. D. Curtin, H. Ishwaran, A. A. Mancuso, *et al.* Comparison of CT and MR imaging in staging of neck metastases. *Radiology* **207** (1998), 123–130.

21. M. Becker, P. Zbären, H. Laeng, *et al.* Neoplastic invasion of the laryngeal cartilage. Comparison of MR imaging and CT with histopathologic correlation. *Radiology* **194** (1995), 661–669.

5

Oral cavity and oropharyngeal cancer

Lawrence E. Ginsberg

Introduction

Malignant tumors of the oral cavity and oropharynx are among the most common head and neck malignancies. Although many of these malignancies are clinically evident, others are not. In other cases, the patient presents with nodal metastases, and imaging is used to detect a primary cancer. In either case, imaging plays an integral role in the staging evaluation of these patients, as well as in their post-treatment work-up [1–3]. This chapter will review the spectrum of imaging findings for malignant tumors of the oral cavity and oropharynx. The focus will be on the initial imaging evaluation, not post-treatment. Imaging of cervical lymph-adenopathy will be covered in Chapter 7.

Choice of modality and technique

The choice of the most appropriate imaging modality remains controversial, or at least influenced by regional and institutional preferences. In some centers, imaging of the oral cavity and oropharynx is conducted primarily with magnetic resonance imaging (MRI) [4]. The emergence of position emission tomography (PET) and PET linked with computed tomography (CT) has changed that equation somewhat, but at the moment, few would argue that PET/CT should be the sole imaging modality for these lesions [5,6]. However, in our institution, unless there is a contrast allergy or renal dysfunction preventing the use of iodinated contrast material, it is our preference to use CT. This preference is based on the consistent and reproducible high-quality images that can be expected from CT, its relatively lower cost and short acquisition time and, with newer, multidetector scanners (MDCT), the availability of multiplanar images. In this choice, we acknowledge that, because of inherent limitations of the technology, as well as the common problem of dental artefact, CT will not show every lesion, particularly those that are

Squamous Cell Cancer of the Neck, ed. Robert Hermans. Published by Cambridge University Press.
© R. Hermans 2009.

superficial or small. Of course, it is precisely those lesions that are generally apparent to the clinician.

Proper CT technique includes slices that are thin, preferably no larger than 1.25 mm; this ensures that reconstructed images can be generated in orthogonal planes with MDCT, if desired. Coronal images are particularly useful for evaluation of lesions in the palate. Another technical consideration is angling around the dental fillings. While some areas (dorsal tongue surface, for instance) may be unavoidably degraded by dental artefact, other areas can be imaged by doing a second series of images through the oral cavity at an angle away from the first set of images. This can be accomplished in different ways, but Fig. 5.1 depicts how this is done at the M. D. Anderson Cancer Center. We image perpendicular to the table-top from thoracic inlet to the top of the orbits, and then we change the gantry angle and take further images through the oral cavity. In this way, lesions that might have been missed in the first pass may become visible on the second. This may visualize not only potential primary sites, such as the floor of mouth, portions of the tongue and pharynx, but also nodal lesions in the upper internal jugular region, lateral retropharyngeal group and parotid gland. One final technical consideration is the "puff-cheek," which will be mentioned in conjunction with oral cavity tumors, below.

Despite our preference for CT, it is understood that occasionally, because of clinician preference, inadvertent ordering of MRI or contraindication to iodinated contrast, some patients with tumors of the oral cavity and oropharynx will be assessed with MRI. For this reason, the radiologist must be familiar with their imaging appearance, and some MRI examples will be interspersed throughout this chapter. Of course, MRI is the preferred modality for the detection of perineural tumor spread, and, as will be mentioned, it may be indicated as a complimentary study if perineural spread is suspected clinically or by CT.

Oral cavity

Subsites of the oral cavity include the oral tongue, gingiva and alveolar ridges, floor of mouth, buccal mucosa, hard palate, lips and retromolar triangle. While each has certain specific imaging features, there are general similarities as well as limitations. Small or superficial lesions, those with little or no bulk unless they enhance prominently, may be invisible on imaging. Since enhancement is variable, we are not able to see every lesion. Fortunately, such lesions are generally visible to the examining physician, who in any case is imaging for other reasons. Those reasons

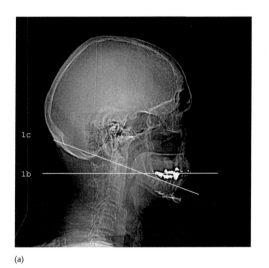

(a)

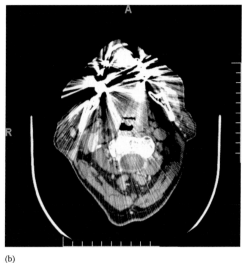

(b)

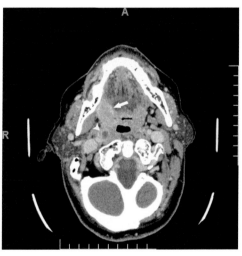

(c)

Fig. 5.1. Value of angling around the dental fillings. (a) A lateral CT scout image. (b) The axial CT image corresponding to the line marked 1b in part (a), directly through the plane of the dental fillings, is essentially uninterpretable. (c) The axial CT image corresponding to the line marked 1c in part (a) was obtained in a separate acquisition, with a gantry angulation that avoided the dental fillings, thus allowing visualization of a right-sided tonsil carcinoma (arrow), as well as a necrotic lateral retropharyngeal nodal metastasis (arrowhead). This type of double acquisition is important in accurate diagnosis of oral cavity, oropharynx and parotid/upper neck masses.

include submucosal extension, bone involvement (for those primary sites [e.g., hard palate or floor of mouth] that are adjacent to bone, images must be reconstructed using a bone algorithm), perineural tumor spread or occult nodal disease. The staging for squamous cell carcinoma of the oral cavity can be found in Table 5.1. Imaging staging can be inaccurate if the lesion cannot be seen in its entirety. For this reason, it is appropriate to mention the stage in the report only when features are clearly identified that would increase the stage of the tumor relative to that defined

Table 5.1. Tumor-staging of lip and oral cavity cancer

Stage	Description
Tis	Carcinoma in situ
T1	Tumor < 2 cm in greatest dimension
T2	Tumor > 2 cm but < 4 cm in greatest dimension
T3	Tumor > 4 cm in greatest dimension
T4a	Lip: tumor invades through cortical bone, inferior alveolar nerve, floor of mouth or skin of face (chin or nose)
	Oral cavity: tumor invades through cortical bone, into deep/extrinsic muscle of tongue (genioglossus, hyoglossus, palatoglossus and styloglossus), maxillary sinus or skin of face
T4b	Lip and oral cavity: tumor invades masticator space, pterygoid plates or skull base, or encases internal carotid artery

From Sobin and Wittekind [7].

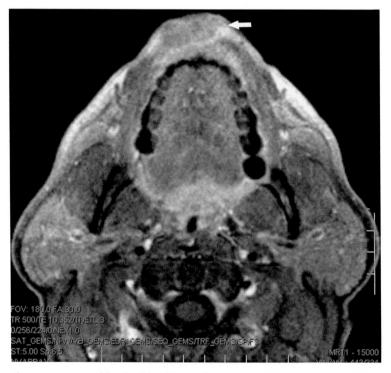

Fig. 5.2. A 42-year-old male with submucosal squamous cell carcinoma of the right lower lip.
Post-contrast fat-suppressed T_1-weighted MRI demonstrates a mass lesion in the right lower lip (arrow). It is important in such cases to exclude perineural tumor spread into the mental foramen and along the more proximal aspects of the mandibular division of the trigeminal nerve; none was present in this case.

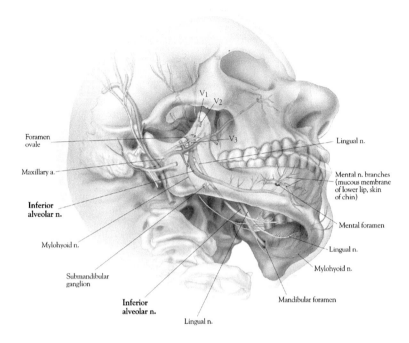

Fig. 5.3. Illustration of mandibular and inferior alveolar nerves. n, nerve; a, artery.

in the clinical examination, or if there is unequivocal imaging evidence of T4 disease (e.g. bone destruction).

Lip

Cancers of the lip are generally visible to the examining physician. Imaging serves to evaluate for submucosal extension (Fig. 5.2) and confirm the extent of disease and nodal involvement; in cancers of the lower lip, imaging will assess for perineural spread along the mental nerve [8, 9]. The mental nerve is the terminal branch of the inferior alveolar branch of the mandibular division of the trigeminal nerve (Fig. 5.3). For cancers of the lower lip, the radiologist must examine the entire course of this nerve, including the mental foramen (on bone windows), the mandibular foramen (on bone and soft-tissue windows), the upper masticator space, the foramen ovale and Meckel's cave (Fig. 5.4). It should be remembered that lower lip cancers may recur in the mental/inferior alveolar nerve with or without imaging or clinical evidence of disease at the primary site. Although our preference is for CT, and CT is quite capable of demonstrating perineural tumor spread, such spread is better seen with MRI [9].

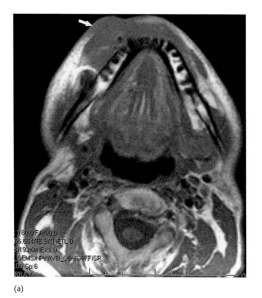

(a)

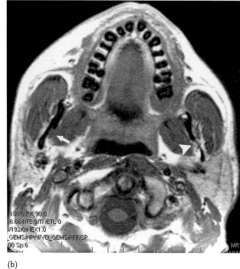

(b)

(c)

Fig. 5.4. A 43-year-old male with recurrent squamous cell carcinoma of the right lower lip, and V$_3$ neuropathy. (a) Axial T$_1$-weighted MRI shows the local recurrence in the lower lip (arrow). (b) Axial pre-contrast T$_1$-weighted MRI shows loss of normal T$_1$ fat signal at the level of the mandibular foramen (arrow), representing perineural tumor spread to at least that level. This tumor first spread from the lip to the mental nerve (see Fig. 5.3). The arrowhead shows normal hyperintense fat in the left mandibular foramen. (c) Coronal post-contrast, fat-suppressed T$_1$-weighted image demonstrates retrograde spread of tumor (arrows) extending from the mandible toward foramen ovale (arrowhead).

Gingiva, alveolar ridge and buccal mucosa

Cancers of the gingiva, generally squamous cell carcinomas, may affect the outer or buccal gingiva, the inner or lingual gingiva, the gingiva along the dentition, or the alveolar ridge, and may be upper or maxillary, or lower–mandibular in origin. Superiorly or inferiorly, buccal gingival cancers may blend with the buccal

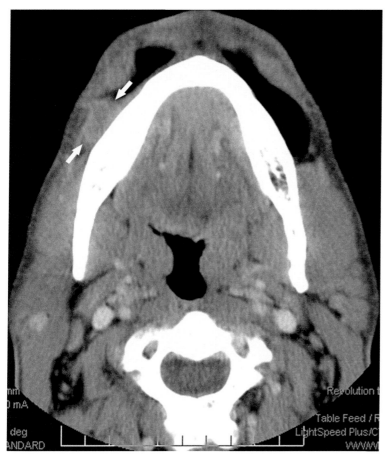

Fig. 5.5. A 48-year-old male with submucosal squamous cell carcinoma of the mandibular gingival and gingivobuccal sulcus. Axial contrast-enhanced CT shows a mass (arrow), made more conspicuous by the "puff cheek" technique of inflating the oral cavity with air to separate the buccal and gingival mucosal surfaces.

mucosa at the gingivobuccal sulcus (Fig. 5.5). The gingivobuccal sulcus is at risk for cancers in so-called "snuff" dippers, or users of chewing tobacco [10]. Lesions in these regions may be difficult to see if small or superficial, or if dental fillings cause image-degrading artefact. Nonetheless many such lesions are visible, especially if the so-called "puff-cheek" technique is employed, whereby the patient is instructed to blow out their cheeks during scanning, which serves to separate the buccal and gingival surfaces, thus allowing better distinction of lesions and their site of origin [11,12] (Fig. 5.5). These lesions are generally seen as masses with variable

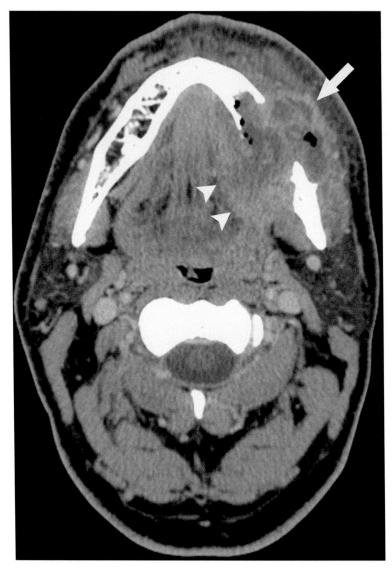

Fig. 5.6. A 52-year-old male with advanced squamous cell carcinoma of the mandibular alveolar ridge. An axial post-contrast CT, soft-tissue window, reveals a massive tumor centered in the left mandibular alveolar ridge, causing extensive bone destruction. There are areas of extension both laterally into the gingivobuccal sulcus (arrow), and medially into the lingual gingiva and floor of mouth (arrowheads). This lesion is stage T4 by virtue of bone destruction.

enhancement. Lesions of the inner or lingual mandibular gingiva may extend to the floor of mouth (Fig. 5.6). Lesions of the lingual maxillary gingiva may spread to the adjacent hard palate. For gingival lesions, the adjacent bone must be scrutinized on bone windows to exclude invasion, which increases the stage to T4. Buccal

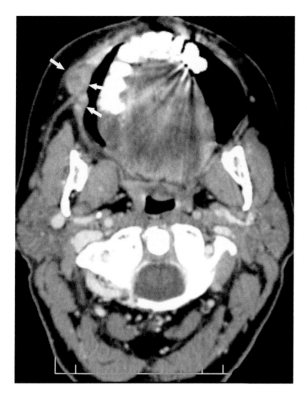

Fig. 5.7. A 65-year-old female with squamous cell carcinoma of the buccal mucosa. Axial post-contrast CT image, also utilizing the puff-cheek technique, shows an infiltrative mass in the right buccal mucosa (arrows).

lesions may be limited to the buccal region (Fig. 5.7) or may extend to involve the contiguous retromolar trigone.

Retromolar trigone

The mucosa behind the last mandibular molar, on the anterior surface of the mandibular ramus, is the retromolar triangle. This region is contiguous laterally with the buccal mucosa and medially with the mucosa of the oropharynx, from or to which cancers of either may spread. Cancers of the retromolar triangle may also invade the ramus, which must be examined with CT bone windows (Fig. 5.8). Malignancies may also extend submucosally to invade the masticator space [13]. The invasion may be flagrant but may in some cases be quite subtle on CT (Fig. 5.9). Invasion of the mandible and/or masticator space can result in mandibular nerve (V$_3$) neuropathy and may have significant implications for resectability and prognosis; if suspected, MRI is indicated [14] (Fig. 5.9).

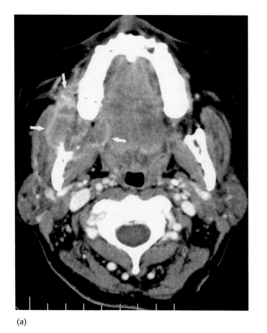

(a)

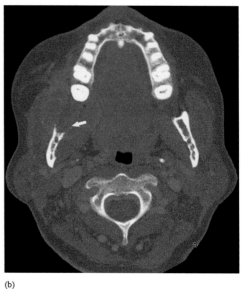

(b)

Fig. 5.8. A 57-year-old woman with squamous cell carcinoma of the right retromolar trigone. (a) Axial post-contrast CT image shows a large, minimally, enhancing, almost rim-enhancing, mass centered in the right retromolar trigone (arrows). (b) Axial CT bone window shows destruction of the anterior aspect of the mandibular ramus (arrow), indicating T4 disease.

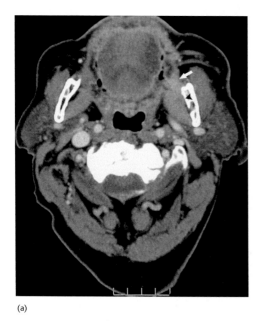

(a)

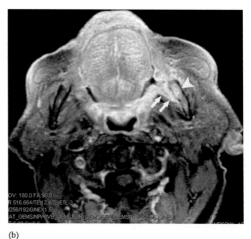

(b)

Fig. 5.9. An 83-year-old man with squamous cell carcinoma of the retromolar trigone and occasional ipsilateral tongue numbness. (a) Axial contrast-enhanced CT partially shows the primary lesion (arrow) but note the subtle effacement or loss of fat plane between the pterygoid musculature and the medial surface of the ramus (arrowhead). This raised the suspicion of extension into the masticator space despite normal bone window (not shown). (b) Axial post-contrast, fat-suppressed T_1-weighted MRI through the mandible shows obvious enhancing tumor between the pterygoid muscles and the anterior ramus (arrows), as well as abnormal enhancement representing tumor within the ramus itself (arrowhead).

Floor of mouth

As already mentioned, the floor of mouth is contiguous with the lingual gingiva, from or to which cancers may spread. Cancers of the floor of mouth are common, though early lesions can be difficult if not impossible to see at imaging. Tumors of the floor of the mouth may also obstruct either the sublingual gland or, more commonly, the submandibular gland; consequently, when the primary lesion itself is difficult to see, its presence may nevertheless be inferred if these salivary glands are obstructed in the absence of a calculus. It should also be noted that an obstructed submandibular gland may be palpable, and clinically regarded as a nodal metastasis. This can provide the radiologist the rare opportunity to downstage the neck by confirming that a palpable mass is an obstructed submandibular gland and not a nodal metastasis.

Radiological evaluation of floor of mouth carcinoma requires the exclusion of bony involvement [13], though it should be kept in mind that some bone may need

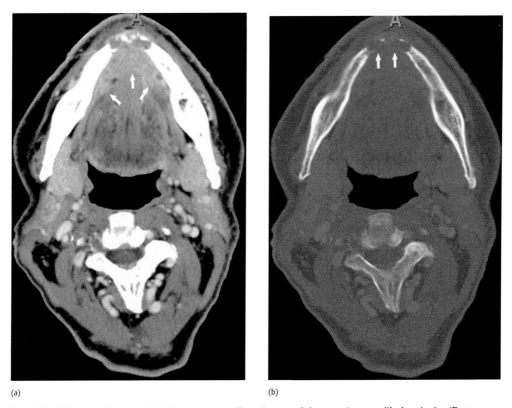

(a)   (b)

Fig. 5.10. A 74-year-old man with T4 squamous cell carcinoma of the anterior mandibular gingiva/floor of mouth. (a) Axial soft-tissue post-contrast CT shows an enhancing mass in the midline floor of mouth (arrows). (b) A CT bone window shows destruction of the mandible (arrows).

to be resected even if not involved (e.g., lingual corticectomy) in order to ensure negative tumor margins. Bone involvement occurs when tumor extends to the adjacent mandibular gingiva (Fig. 5.10) and, of course, indicates T4 disease. Deep submucosal extension can involve the sublingual space (the region bounded

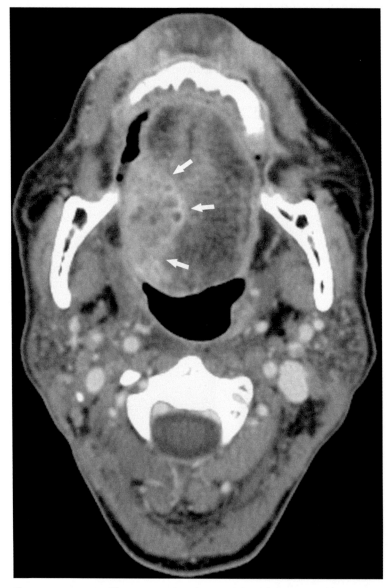

Fig. 5.11. A 53-year-old woman previously treated for soft palate carcinoma, now with new primary cancer of the right oral tongue. Axial CT shows an enhancing mass in the right mid-posterior oral tongue (arrows).

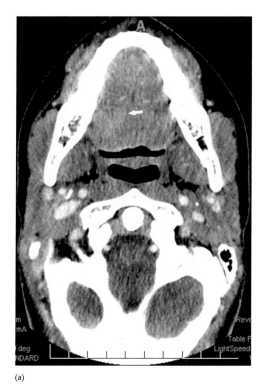
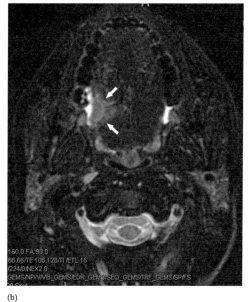

(a)   (b)

Fig. 5.12. A 19-year-old woman with squamous cell carcinoma of the right posterior oral tongue.
(a) Axial post-contrast CT shows only a faintly visible lesion in the right posterolateral tongue (arrow).
(b) Axial T$_2$-weighted MRI shows the lesion more clearly (arrows).

laterally by the mylohyoid muscle and medially by the genioglosssus/geniohyoid muscle bellies), which contains the neurovascular bundle of the tongue [13]. Such involvement is a poor prognostic indicator, and it may cause hypoglossal denervation [14]. Some floor of mouth lesions achieve dramatic size and are quite destructive at diagnosis. In such cases, the precise site of origin may be indeterminate.

Oral tongue

Cancers of the oral, or anterior two thirds of the tongue are very common in a busy head and neck cancer service. On contrast-enhanced CT, these lesions are generally evident as areas of abnormal enhancement (Fig. 5.11) unless the lesion is too small to be seen. Oral tongue lesions are often obscured by dental artefact but can sometimes be seen at a different gantry angulation, as already mentioned; some

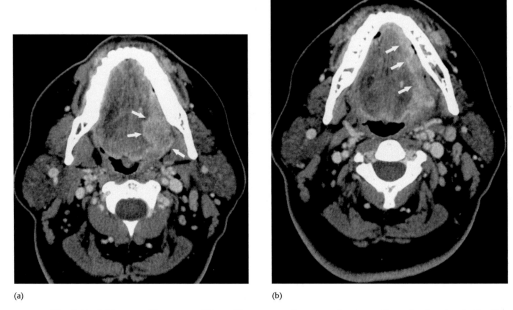

(a)   (b)

Fig. 5.13. A 39-year-old woman with oral tongue carcinoma and a suggestion of extension to the floor of mouth. (a) Axial post-contrast CT shows an obvious enhancing mass in the left lateral oral tongue (arrows). (b) At a more inferior level, imaging shows the suggestion of extension to the left floor of mouth (arrows), but the floor of mouth was uninvolved clinically and at surgery. This was probably a tumor along the lateral and perhaps ventral tongue surface, but radiographically was inseparable from the floor of mouth.

lesions with MRI can also be seen more readily (Fig. 5.12). Magnetic resonance is itself a good imaging modality for staging tongue carcinoma. Cancers of the tongue, indeed of all oral cavity and oropharyngeal cancers, appear as a low signal on T_1-weighted images, and a high signal on T_2-weighted images; they enhance with gadolinium [15] (Fig. 5.12). The radiologist must check for deep invasion that involves the floor of mouth, and subclinical extension across the midline, which may have surgical implications [13]. While extension to the floor of the mouth is sometimes obvious, the ventral tongue surface is immediately adjacent to the floor of the mouth in a closed mouth and, consequently, axial plane imaging cannot always reveal tumor extension between these two structures (Fig. 5.13).

Hard palate

The hard palate is not frequently involved with cancer, but when it is, by virtue of its high concentration of minor salivary glands, it has a greater likelihood of having

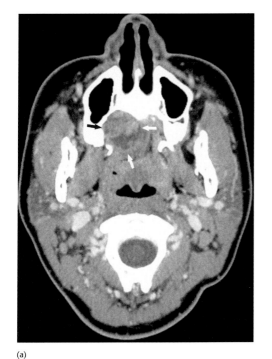
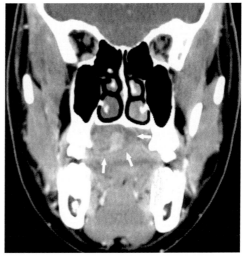

(a)   (b)

**Fig. 5.14. A 25-year-old man with pleomorphic adenoma of the hard palate. Axial (a) and coronal
(b) reconstructed post-contrast CT images show a slightly heterogeneous, basically non-enhancing mass in
the right hard palate (arrows). There was no bone destruction. The imaging here is non-specific (see Fig. 5.15).**

non-squamous cell histology [16]. Salivary malignancies, as well as benign salivary
neoplasms, must be considered in the differential diagnosis when hard palate
tumors are encountered (Fig. 5.14). Adjacent mucosal surfaces from or to which
palate cancers may spread include the maxillary alveolar ridge/lingua gingiva and
soft palate. Radiographically, these lesions are similar to other oral cavity lesions,
but there are some specific considerations. Because of its horizontal orientation, the
palate lends itself quite well to imaging in the coronal and sagittal planes, and
indeed such views are critical in completely evaluating hard palate lesions, as some
lesions may be invisible, or nearly so, in the axial plane (Fig. 5.14). Obviously, given
the bony nature of the hard palate, bone windows must also be assessed. Generally,
but not always, malignancy may be suggested by the presence of bony destruction or
other signs of malignancy, but this is not always true as non-destructive lesions may
still be low-grade malignancies such as mucoepidermoid carcinoma (Fig. 5.15).
Obviously, destructive lesions suggest aggressive malignancy (Fig. 5.16).

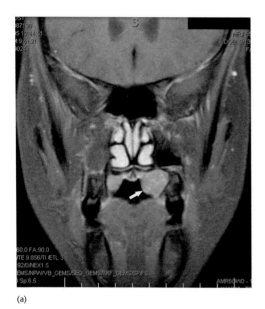
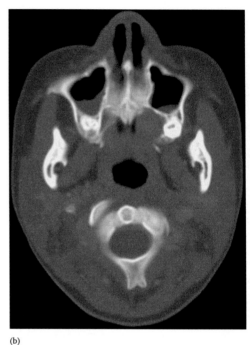

(a)   (b)

Fig. 5.15. A hard palate mucoepidermoid carcinoma in a 16-year-old woman. (a) Coronal post-contrast, fat-suppressed T$_1$-weighted MRI shows a mildly enhancing mass in the left hard palate (arrow). (b) The axial CT bone window shows some non-destructive remodeling, and is, therefore, non-specific. Note the similarity between this tumor and that shown in Fig. 5.14.

Perineural spread is another concern in hard palate malignancies, because the palatine branches of the maxillary division of the trigeminal nerve provide a ready route for spread up to the pterygopalatine fossa [16] (Fig. 5.17). In fact, minor salivary malignancies of hard palate origin may be entirely submucosal and thus clinically silent, and they may actually spread perineurally prior to their detection [16]. For this reason, not only must any known hard palate cancer have radiological assessment of the entire course of the maxillary nerve up to the cavernous sinus, but any patient presenting with an unexplained lesion in the cavernous sinus or pterygopalatine fossa, or trigeminal neuropathy, must have their palates scrutinized for a possible occult malignancy. In particular, the greater palatine foramen should be examined on CT bone windows for evidence of widening, a sign of perineural spread (or possibly direct tumor invasion) (Fig. 5.18). Finally, inasmuch as MRI is the best imaging procedure for the evaluation of perineural spread, the case can be made for its choice as the main imaging modality for hard palate lesions.

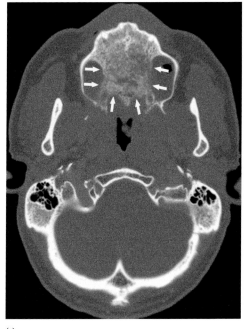

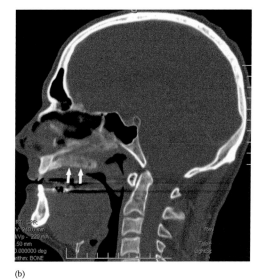

(a)

(b)

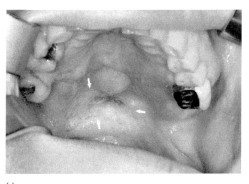

(c)

Fig. 5.16. A 46-year-old man with invasive hard palate squamous cell carcinoma. (a,b) Axial (a) and sagittal (b) reconstructed CT bone window images show a permeative destruction of the hard palate (arrows). (c) A gross photograph showing the ulcerative lesion of the posterior hard palate (arrows). Much of the lesion was submucosal. (Part (c) is available in color in the plate section.)

Oropharynx

Subsites of the oropharynx include the base of tongue and vallecula, the tonsil and pharyngeal walls, and the soft palate. Collectively, these are among the most common sites of malignancy in the head and neck. While squamous cell carcinoma is far and away the most likely histological subtype, as well as the minor salivary gland malignancies that can occur anywhere in the upper aerodigestive tract

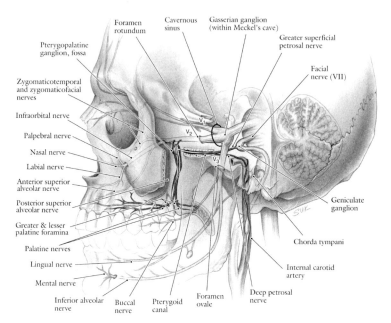

Fig. 5.17. Illustration of trigeminal nerve anatomy relevant to perineural spread from the palate.

mucosa, the tonsils and tongue base, by virtue of their lymphoid content, can also give rise to lymphomas; the imaging appearance for these tumors are generally indistinguishable from one another. The staging for squamous cell carcinoma of the oral cavity can be found in Table 5.2.

Although oropharyngeal cancers are often painful, some are not. Patients with these tumors may present with a neck mass, and only the diagnosis of squamous cell carcinoma in these metastatic lymph nodes will prompt a clinical and/or radiographic search for a primary cancer. Uniquely, oropharyngeal cancers are sometimes associated with completely or predominantly cystic nodal metastases, and while a discussion of nodal disease is not part of the brief of this chapter, it deserves special mention [17]. Such cyst-like nodes are often misinterpreted as benign entities, such as a second branchial cleft cyst; aspiration of such cysts will typically be histologically benign, and thus the offending malignancy may go undetected and untreated [17]. In many of these cases, the oropharyngeal cancer is small or occult either on imaging or clinically, or both. Of course, other nodal metastases, if present, should suggest malignancy and not a benign cyst. Given that branchial cleft cysts usually occur in a younger age group than does oropharyngeal cancer, the radiologist should hesitate before diagnosing an upper internal jugular region cystic

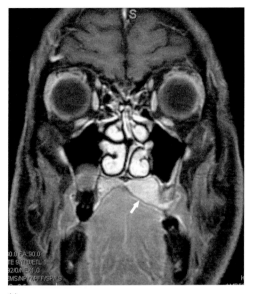

(a)

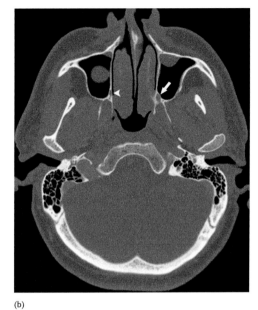

(b)

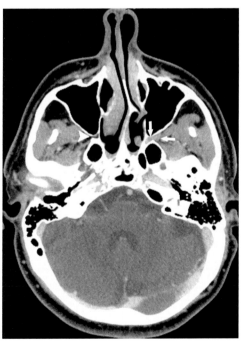

(c)

Fig. 5.18. A 55-year-old man with adenoid cystic carcinoma of the hard palate and perineural tumor spread. (a) Coronal post-contrast, fat-suppressed T_1-weighted MRI shows a moderately enhancing mass in the left hard palate (arrow). (b) Axial bone-window CT shows enlargement of the left greater palatine foramen (arrow). Note the normal right greater palatine foramen (arrowhead). (c) Axial soft-tissue CT image at a higher level shows abnormal enhancement and loss of fat attenuation in the left pterygopalatine fossa (arrows). The normal right pterygopalatine fossa is indicated with an arrowhead. This structure must be scrutinized in any patient with V_2 neuropathy or a cancer along the anatomic distribution of this nerve.

Table 5.2. Tumor staging of oropharyngeal cancer

Stage	Description
Tis	Carcinoma in situ
T1	Tumor $<2\,$cm in greatest dimension
T2	Tumor $>2\,$cm but $<4\,$cm in greatest dimension
T3	Tumor $>4\,$cm in greatest dimension
T4a	Tumor invades any of the following: larynx, deep/extrinsic muscle of the tongue (genioglossus, hyoglossus, palatoglossus and styloglossus), medial pterygoid, hard palate or mandible
T4b	Tumor invades any of the following: lateral pterygoid muscle, pterygoid plates, lateral nasopharynx or skull base, or encases the carotid artery

From Sobin and Wittekind [7].

mass as benign in an older patient, and rather should be very suspicious of oropharyngeal cancer, *even if such a lesion is not apparent on the scan.*

As with lesions described elsewhere in this chapter, small lesions can be invisible on imaging because of their size or obscuring dental artefact on CT. In addition, prominent and/or asymmetric lymphoid tissue in the tongue base/vallecula and tonsils can either mask or mimic tumors. For the most part, oropharyngeal cancers are visible by virtue of their bulk or mass effect, their enhancement or signal abnormality, or both.

Tonsillopharyngeal region

This section is intended to cover lesions restricted to the tonsils as well as those that involve the pharyngeal wall adjacent to but separate from the faucial tonsils, and the posterior pharyngeal wall. The faucial or palatine tonsil is bounded anteriorly by the palatoglossal fold (arch) or anterior pillar, and posteriorly by the palatopharyngeal fold (arch) or posterior pillar. In my experience, though these folds/pillars are readily evident clinically, they are usually difficult to identify on imaging. Consequently, distinction between cancers arising primarily in the tonsil versus those arising in the adjacent pillars can be impossible. What is important is that tonsil cancers can use the pillars as a scaffold with which to spread to adjacent anatomical sites.

Nonetheless, tonsillar cancers run the gamut from small, non-invasive and invisible, or nearly so, on imaging [18] (Fig. 5.19) to massive, invasive and obvious on imaging (Fig. 5.20). In tumors that are difficult to see on CT or MRI, there may be value in performing a PET/CT (Fig. 5.19), although it may be argued that the

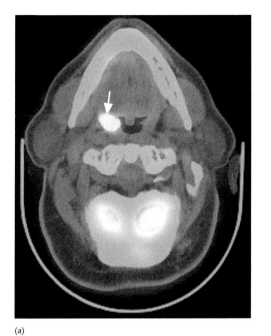

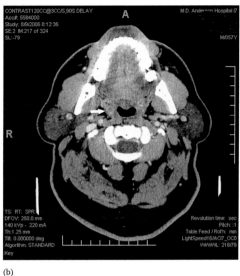

(a)

(b)

Fig. 5.19. Clinically T0 squamous cell carcinoma in a 57-year-old man presenting with neck metastasis. No abnormality was found at physical examination and MR and CT imaging were interpreted as negative. (a) Use of PET–CT shows intense ^{18}F-fluorodeoxyglucose activity in the right tonsil (arrow). This prompted a review of the CT (b), and in retrospect, the tonsillar primary is subtly apparent (arrow).

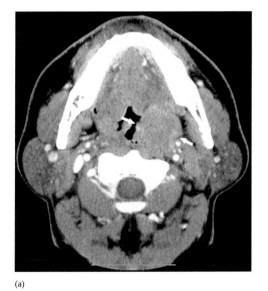

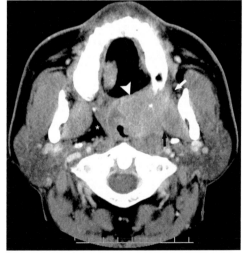

(a)

(b)

Fig. 5.20. A 57-year-old man with extensive oropharyngeal squamous cell carcinoma. (a) The axial CT image through the tonsillar fossa shows a bulky, mildly enhancing mass in the left tonsil (arrows). (b) At a slightly higher level, the image shows involvement of the soft palate (arrowhead) and lateral extension towards the retromolar trigone (white arrow). Note also effacement of the left parapharyngeal space fat, and poor margins between that fat and the masticator muscles (black arrow), indicating invasion. The intact right parapharyngeal fat is indicated with an asterisk.

primary might either be evident clinically or be detectable at examination under anesthesia. It could also be argued that, in any case, the treatment of a presumed small oropharyngeal cancer would be the same regardless.

Tonsillar tumors may spread circumferentially to involve the posterior pharyngeal wall and the contralateral tonsil, superiorly to the soft palate [18] (Fig. 5.20), anteriorly into the tongue base or inferiorly into the hypopharynx, such that the precise site of origin may be impossible to determine. Some areas of spread may be superficial and

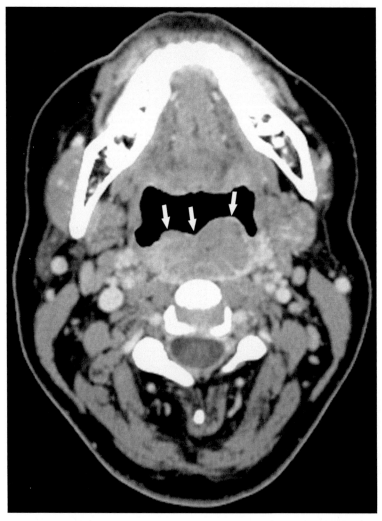

Fig. 5.21. Posterior wall oropharyngeal squamous cell carcinoma in a 44-year-old woman presenting with otalgia, dysphagia and odynophagia. Axial CT image shows a bulky enhancing mass along the posterior pharyngeal wall (arrows).

only visible clinically; others may be submucosal and visible only radiographically. Laterally, tonsillopharyngeal lesions can involve the parapharyngeal or masticator spaces (Fig. 5.20). In addition to tonsil cancers spreading to the posterior pharyngeal wall, they may occur primarily within, and be restricted to, the posterior wall (Fig. 5.21). Such lesions have a tendency to burrow submucosally. This is one of the important roles of imaging oropharyngeal cancer: to detect areas of submucosal spread.

Although it is our preference to image most oropharyngeal cancers with CT, the majority of these lesions are also quite well seen with MRI.

Base of tongue

The tongue base, that area of tongue posterior to the circumvallate papillae and down to the vallecula, bounded laterally by the glossopharyngeal sulcus, is also a very common site of malignancy. As with tonsil cancers, these may be very subtle (Fig. 5.22) or massive and invasive (Fig. 5.23). They may be superficial/exophytic or extend

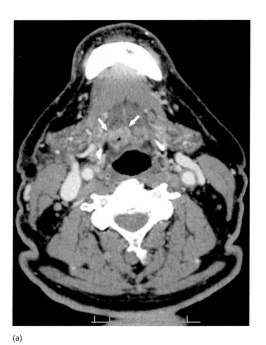
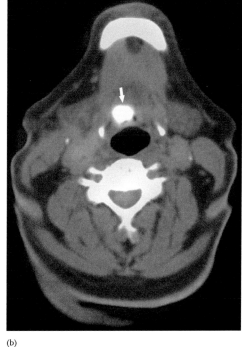

(a) (b)

Fig. 5.22. A subtle vallecular carcinoma in a 65-year-old man presenting with a neck metastasis. (a) Axial CT shows a suggestion of a faintly enhancing mass in the right vallecula (arrows). (b) This lesion was far more convincing on PET–CT (arrow). This cancer was proven at surgery.

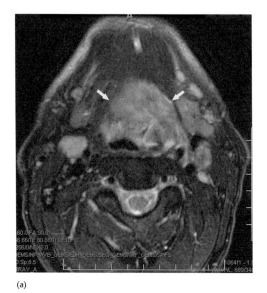

(a)

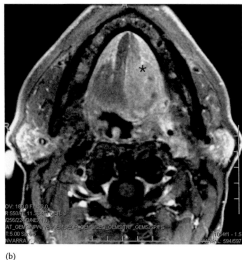

(b)

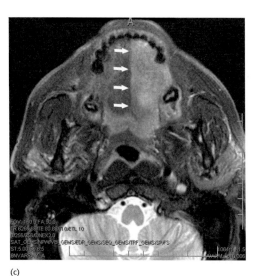

(c)

Fig. 5.23. Advanced base of tongue carcinoma in a 46-year-old man presenting with otalgia and dysphagia, followed by left-sided tongue weakness. (a) Axial T$_2$-weighted MRI shows a hyperintense mass in the tongue base (arrows). Bilateral upper internal jugular nodal metastases are visible. (b) The same sequence at a slightly more superior level demonstrates deep anterior submucosal extension into the sublingual space (asterisk), resulting in hypoglossal paralysis. (c) The T$_2$-weighted MRI shows signal hyperintensity in the left hemitongue, indicating subacute denervation. Note how this respects the midline (arrows).

submucosally. Sites of adjacent spread include anteriorly into the deep oral tongue and floor of mouth (Fig. 5.23), laterally via the glossopharyngeal sulcus into the pharyngeal side wall (Fig. 5.24), and inferiorly into the supraglottic structures (epiglottis and aryepiglottic folds).

The glossopharyngeal sulcus, the junction of the lateral tongue base and pharyngeal wall, deserves special mention. Tumors arise here quite frequently but are

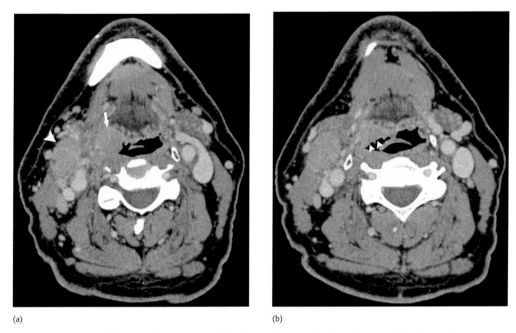

(a)   (b)

Fig. 5.24. A 58-year-old man with carcinoma of the glossopharyngeal sulcus. (a) An axial CT image shows a small, nearly isodense mass in the right glossopharyngeal sulcus (arrow). There is a large right upper internal jugular nodal metastasis (arrowhead). Extension to or from the contiguous tonsil and base of tongue should be evaluated in such cases. (b) Lower down, involvement of the tongue base near the vallecula can be seen (arrowheads).

not neatly categorized as having arisen in either location (Fig. 5.24). Furthermore, such lesions may be quite subtle, almost or completely imperceptible radiologically, and sometimes clinically as well. As with small lesions in any location, cross-sectional imaging alone may be inadequate for imaging diagnosis; in such cases, there may be a role for PET/CT (Figs. 5.19 and 5.22).

Soft palate

Located immediately posterior to the hard palate, the soft palate spreads out laterally in a bat-wing fashion and is contiguous via the pillars with the tongue and pharyngeal wall, and retromolar trigone, and, of course, anteriorly with the hard palate, all of which represent sites to or from which cancers may spread. Relatively few cancers begin in and stay restricted to the soft palate, but they do occur (Fig. 5.25). It is the radiologist's job to detect areas of contiguous spread: mucosally, submucosally or deep spread that may not be detected clinically. In

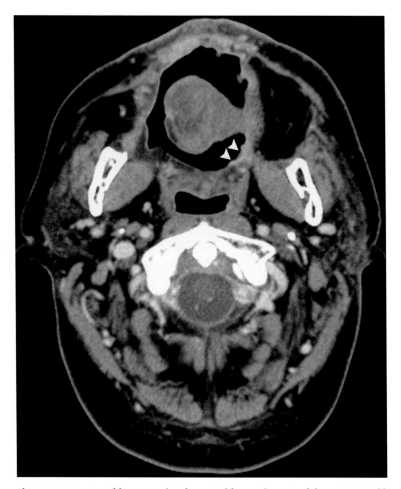

Fig. 5.25. A 61-year-old man previously treated for carcinomas of the tongue and buccal mucosa, now with a third primary cancer of the soft palate. Axial CT image shows a superficial, subtly enhancing lesion on the lingual surface of the soft palate (arrowheads), proven at biopsy to be squamous cell carcinoma.

addition, soft palate cancers may gain access to the palatine branches of the maxillary nerve and, thus, result in perineural spread [16]. The radiologist must, therefore, check the course of the lesser palatine nerves, including the lesser palatine foramen, the pterygopalatine fossa, the foramen rotundum and the cavernous sinus. In terms of imaging, the radiologist may occasionally find the CT scout image useful to observe the enlargement of a soft palate so uniformly infiltrated with tumor that the cross-sectional imaging is difficult to call abnormal.

REFERENCES

1. H. R. Harnsberger, R. H. Wiggins, P. A. Hudgins, *et al. Diagnostic Imaging. Head and Neck*, vol. 1 (Salt Lake City, UT: Amirsys, 2004), various pages.

2. S. K. Mukherji, J. Castelijns, M. Castillo. Squamous cell carcinoma of the oropharynx and oral cavity: How imaging makes a difference. *Semin Ultrasound, CT MRI* **19** (1998), 463–475.

3. S. K. Mukherji, H. R. Pillsbury, M. Castillo. Imaging squamous cell carcinomas of the upper aerodigestive tract: what clinicians need to know. *Radiology* **205** (1997), 629–646.

4. E. Wiener, C. Pautke, T. M. Link, A. Neff, A. Kolk. Comparison of 16-slice MSCT and MRI in the assessment of squamous cell carcinoma of the oral cavity. *Eur J Radiol* **58** (2006), 113–118.

5. F. Dammann, M. Horger, M. Mueller-Berg, *et al.* Rational diagnosis of squamous cell carcinoma of the head and neck region: comparative evaluation of CT, MRI, and 18FDG PET. *Am J Roentgenol* **184** (2005), 1326–1331.

6. S. H. Ng, T. C. Yen, C. T. Liao, *et al.* 18F-FDG PET and CT/MRI in oral cavity squamous cell carcinoma: a prospective study of 124 patients with histologic correlation. *J Nucl Med* **46** (2005), 1136–1143.

7. L. H. Sobin, C. Wittekind (eds.) *UICC TNM Classification of Malignant Tumors*, 6th edn (New York: Wiley-Liss, 2002).

8. L. E. Ginsberg. Imaging of perineural tumor spread in head and neck cancer. In *Head and Neck Imaging*, ed. P. M. Som, H. D. Curtin (St. Louis: Mosby, 2003).

9. L. E. Ginsberg. MR imaging of perineural tumor spread. *Neuroimaging Clin North Am* **14** (2004), 663–677.

10. D. M. Winn, W. J. Blot, C. M. Shy, *et al.* Snuff dipping and oral cancer among women in the southern United States. *N Engl J Med* **304** (1981), 745–749.

11. J. L. Weissman, R. L. Carrau. "Puffed-cheek" CT improves evaluation of the oral cavity. *Am J Neuroradiol* **22** (2001), 741–744.

12. G. M. Fatterpekar, B. N. Delman, M. M. Shroff, *et al.* Distension technique to improve computed tomographic evaluation of oral cavity lesions. *Arch Otolaryngol Head Neck Surg* **129** (2003), 229–232.

13. W. R. K. Smoker. The oral cavity. In *Head and Neck Imaging*, ed. P. M. Som, H. D. Curtin (St. Louis: Mosby, 2003), pp. 1377–1464.

14. S. K. Mukherji, S. M. Weeks, M. Castillo, *et al.* Squamous cell carcinomas that arise in the oral cavity and tongue base: can CT help predict perineural or vascular invasion? *Radiology* **198** (1996), 157–162.

15. C. Kirsch. Oral cavity cancer. *Top Magn Reson Imaging* **18** (2007), 269–280.

16. L. E. Ginsberg, F. Demonte. Palatal adenoid cystic carcinoma presenting as perineural spread to the cavernous sinus. *Skull Base Surg* **8** (1998), 39–43.

17. D. Goldenber, J. Scuibba, W. M. Koch. Cystic metastasis from head and neck squamous cell cancer: a distinct disease variant? *Head Neck* **28** (2006), 633–638.

18. H. E. Stambuk, S. Karimi, N. Lee, S. G. Patel. Oral cavity and oropharynx tumors. *Radiol Clin North Am* **45** (2007), 1–20.

6

Nasopharyngeal cancer

Vincent F. H. Chong

Introduction

Nasopharyngeal carcinoma (NPC) is a unique malignancy showing a distinct racial and geographical distribution. The annual incidence rate (per 100 000 per year) in 1988–1992 ranged from < 1 among Caucasians to > 20 among southern Chinese male populations [1]. The highest incidence rates are found in southern Chinese and this pattern persists in those who have emigrated. The incidence in high-risk populations rises after 30 years of age, peaks at 40–60 years and declines thereafter. This malignancy is more common in males, with a male to female ratio of 2.5:1. The time trend in the past was generally stable in most populations, but in recent years a gradual decline has been noted.

The etiology is based on the outcome of the interaction among genetic suscept-ibility, environmental factors (including chemical carcinogens) and the Epstein–Barr virus (EBV) [2,3].

Anatomy of the nasopharynx

The nasopharynx is a fibromuscular sling hanging from the skull base. Its shape and volume resembles the terminal segments of the thumb. The sphenoid sinus and the basisphenoid form the roof of the nasopharynx (Fig. 6.1). The roof slopes poster-iorly, with the basiocciput, atlas and axis forming the posterior wall. Anteriorly, it is contiguous with the choanae, with the posterior nasal margin forming the anterior limit. The lateral nasopharynx wall is formed from front to back by the medial pterygoid plate, the palatal muscles, the torus tubarius and the lateral pharyngeal recess (fossa of Rosenmuller). The soft palate separates the nasopharynx from the oropharynx.

The stiff pharyngobasilar fascia maintains the shape of the nasopharynx. This tough aponeurosis is the cranial extension of the superior constrictor muscle from

Squamous Cell Cancer of the Neck, ed. Robert Hermans. Published by Cambridge University Press.
© R. Hermans 2009.

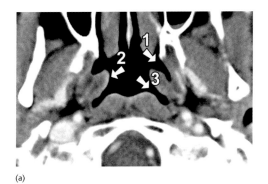 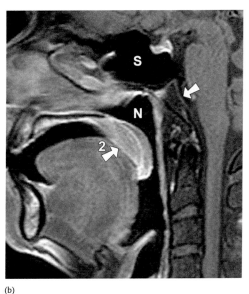

(a)   (b)

Fig. 6.1. Normal anatomy of the nasopharynx. (a) Axial CT shows the left eustachian tube opening (arrow 1), torus tubarius (arrow 2) and fossa of Rosenmuller (arrow 3). (b) Sagittal T_1-weighted MRI (different patient) shows the nasopharynx (N), sphenoid sinus (S), clivus (arrow) and soft palate (arrow 2).

the level of the soft palate to the base of the skull. This fascia demarcates the nasopharynx within and the parapharyngeal tissues without.

The adenoids occupy the roof of the nasopharynx. They decrease in volume with age but may persist as tags of tissue into adulthood. Residual lymphoid tissue may occasionally mimic neoplasms on imaging studies. Computed tomography (CT) and magnetic resonance imaging (MRI) with T_1-weighted images cannot separate lymphoid tissues from the underlying muscles. However, T_2-weighted MRI show good contrast between the high signal intensity of lymphoid tissue and the low signal intensity of muscles. Lymphoid tissues are located superficially and never penetrate the underlying muscle.

The eustachian tube enters the nasopharynx through an opening in the pharyngobasilar fascia, called the sinus of Morgagni. The pharyngeal end of the eustachian tube, composed of cartilage, protrudes in the pharyngeal lumen and is called the torus tubarius.

The fossa of Rosenmuller is located superior and posterior to the torus tubarius. The inverted J-configuration of the torus tubarius results in the fossa appearing posterior (on axial images) and superior (on coronal images) to the eustachian tube orifice. This recess is formed by the mucosal reflection over the longus colli muscle and the inner side of the torus tubarius.

The parapharyngeal space (PPS) separates the wall of the nasopharyngeal mucosa from the masticator space. The PPS extends from the skull base to the oropharynx and consists of a loose network of fibrofatty tissue. A NPC frequently extends across the PPS and infiltrates the muscles of mastication [4]. This may result in trismus or perineural infiltration of the mandibular nerve. The carotid space is located behind the PPS and forms the posterior most lateral compartment of the nasopharynx. Between the nasopharynx and the vertebral bodies is the retropharyngeal space. Within this space are the lateral retropharyngeal (LRP) nodes, which form the first echelon nodes in the lymphatic drainage of the nasopharynx.

Superolateral to the fossa of Rosenmuller, and within the pharyngobasilar fascia, is the foramen lacerum. This foramen is formed by the posterior margin of the petrous apex and the upper clivus. The inferior portion of this opening is filled with cartilage. The carotid artery enters the carotid canal and runs over the superior portion of the foramen lacerum before emerging into the middle cranial fossa. Lateral to the foramen lacerum, and outside the pharyngobasilar fascia, is the foramen ovale. It transmits the mandibular nerve, which innervates the muscles of mastication.

Pathological anatomy and imaging

Most NPC originates in the fossa of Rosenmuller (Fig. 6.2). Tumors tend to spread submucosally, with early infiltration of the palatal muscles, in particular the levator veli palatini. As this muscle is responsible for opening the eustachian tube orifice during swallowing, dysfunction leads to disequilibrium in the air pressure within the middle ear and the nasopharynx. The eustachian tube orifice may also be obstructed by the tumor itself. These factors commonly result in serous otitis media [5]. Extension of the PPS may also affect tubal function [6]. When NPC extends outside the nasopharynx, it spreads along a well-defined route [7,8]. Accurate staging can be performed by mapping disease extent according to the TNM staging system (Tables 6.1 and 6.2) [9]. The following patterns of spread may be seen in various combinations.

Anterior spread

Tumors often spread anteriorly into the nasal fossa and may infiltrate the pterygopalatine fossa (PPF) through the sphenopalatine foramen [10]. The earliest sign of involvement of the PPF is obliteration of the normal fat content. This can be readily

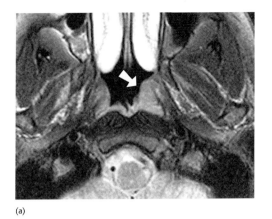
(a)

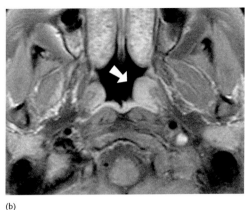
(b)

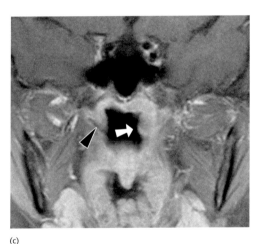
(c)

**Fig. 6.2. Early nasopharyngeal carcinoma.
(a) Axial T₂-weighted MRI shows an early
tumor with high signal intensity in the left
fossa of Rosenmuller (arrow). (b) Axial
contrast-enhanced MRI shows tumor
enhancement. Tumor (arrow) is confined to the
mucosa with no extension into the deeper
structures. (c) Coronal-contrast enhanced MRI
shows tumor (arrow) originating in the left
fossa. Note the normal right fossa of
Rosenmuller (arrowhead).**

seen on CT and MRI. Once the tumor is in the PPF, the maxillary nerve is at risk
(Fig 6.3). Perineural spread can extend into the intracranial cavity through the
foramen rotundum [11]. The tumor can infiltrate further superiorly into the inferior
orbital fissure and subsequently extend into the orbital apex. From the orbital apex,
the tumor can extend intracranially through the superior orbital fissure (Fig. 6.4).

Lateral spread

Lateral spread (the most common direction) results in PPS infiltration. This can be
recognized by the partial or complete effacement of the fat-filled PPS (Fig. 6.5). The
mandibular nerve is located in the masticator space, close to the PPS. Hence tumor
spreading laterally may result in perineural infiltration and subsequent intracranial

Table 6.1. Staging of nasopharyngeal carcinoma

Stage	Description
T: primary tumor	
T1	Tumor confined to nasopharynx
T2	Tumor extends to soft tissue of oropharynx and/or nasal fossa
T2a	Without parapharyngeal extension
T2b	With parapharyngeal extension
T3	Tumor invades bony structures and/or paranasal sinuses
T4	Tumor with intracranial extension and/or involvement of cranial nerves, infratemporal fossa, hypopharynx, or orbit
N: regional lymph nodes	
NX	Regional lymph nodes cannot be assessed
N0	No regional lymph node metastasis
N1	Unilateral metastasis in lymph node(s), < 6 cm or less in greatest dimension, above supraclavicular fossa
N2	Bilateral metastasis in lymph node(s), < 6 cm or less in greatest dimension, above supraclavicular fossa
N3	Metastasis in lymph node(s): > 6 cm in dimension and or in the supraclavicular fossa

From Greene *et al.* [9].

Table 6.2. Nasopharyngeal carcinoma: stage grouping

Stage	Tumor	Node	Metastases
0	Tis	N0	M0
I	T1	N0	M0
IIA	T2a	N0	M0
IIB	T1	N1	M0
	T2a	N1	M0
	T2b	N0, N1	M0
III	T1	N2	M0
	T2a, T2b	N2	M0
	T3	N0, N1, N2	M0
IVA	T4	N0, N1, N2	M0
IVB	Any T	N3	M0
IVC	Any T	Any N	M1

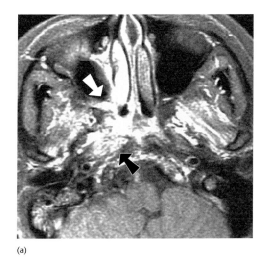

(a)

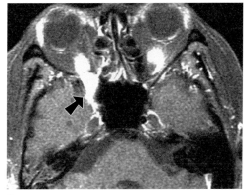

(b)

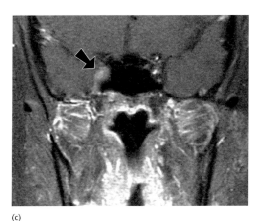

(c)

Fig. 6.3. Nasopharyngeal carcinoma with infiltration of the pterygopalatine fossa and maxillary nerve. (a) Axial contrast-enhanced MRI shows tumor in the nasopharynx (black arrow) with extension into the right pterygopalatine fossa (white arrow). (b) Axial contrast-enhanced MRI shows tumor extending through the right foramen rotundum into the cavernous sinus (arrow). (c) Coronal contrast-enhanced MRI shows thickening and increased enhancement of the cavernous sinus (arrow).

extension. When the medial or lateral pterygoid muscles are infiltrated, the patient may complain of trismus [12]. Posterolateral spread into the retrostyloid compartment may result in the infiltration of the carotid space, placing the last four cranial nerves at risk [13,14].

Posterior spread

When NPC spreads posteriorly, it infiltrates the prevertebral muscles. Destruction of the vertebral bodies and involvement of the spinal canal is occasionally seen in late presentations (Fig. 6.5).

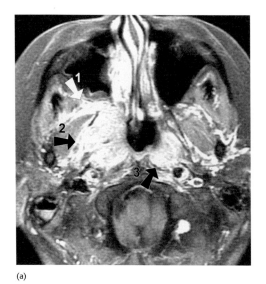

(a)

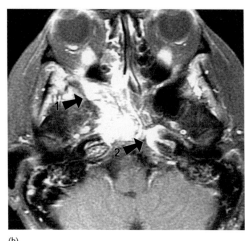

(b)

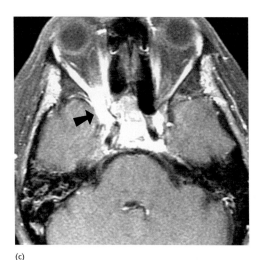

(c)

Fig. 6.4. Extensive nasopharyngeal carcinoma with right-sided orbital apex involvement. (a) Axial contrast-enhanced MRI shows tumor invading the right pterygopalatine fossa (arrow 1) with further extension into right masticator space. Note also tumor extending into the parapharyngeal and masticator spaces (arrow 2). Tumor is also present in the left fossa of Rosenmuller (arrow 3). (b) Axial contrast-enhanced MRI shows tumor extension into the inferior orbital fissure (arrow 1). Note tumor extension into the left foramen lacerum (arrow 2). (c) Axial contrast-enhanced MRI shows tumor infiltration into orbital apex and extension into intracranial cavity via superior orbital fissure (arrow).

Inferior spread

Some tumors show preferential inferior spread. Tumor often extends inferiorly along the submucosal plane and may not be readily appreciated during clinical inspection. Imaging in such instances provides a more accurate means of demonstrating disease extent. Inferior extension into the oropharynx is readily appreciated on coronal and/ or sagittal MRI. However, a diagnosis of oropharyngeal involvement can also be made with confidence on axial sections. In axial images, the oropharynx is deemed involved when tumor can be seen inferior to C1/C2 (Fig. 6.6).

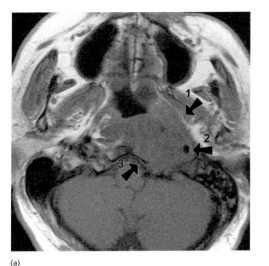
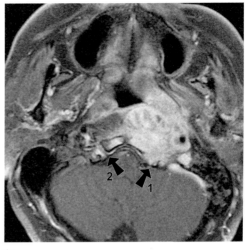

(a)   (b)

Fig. 6.5. Nasopharyngeal carcinoma with lateral and posterior spread. (a) Axial T_1-weighted MRI shows tumor extending laterally to involve the left parapharyngeal space (arrow 1), and posteriorly to encase the carotid sheath (arrow 2). Involvement of the prevertebral space and marrow replacement in the clivus is also seen (arrow 3). (b) Axial contrast-enhanced MRI shows tumor eroding the clivus and involving the left hypoglossal canal with consequent spread into the posterior cranial fossa (arrow 1). Note the normal right hypoglossal canal (arrow 2).

Superior spread

Skull base erosion is detected in up to one third of the patients. The frequency of intracranial spread on CT is > 12% and on MRI 31% [7,15]. For a long time, NPC was believed to have an unimpeded pathway of infiltration into the cranial cavity through the foramen lacerum [16,17]. Studies using CT have suggested that the most common manner of intracranial spread is by direct erosion [18,19].

With the advent of MRI, the most common route of intracranial spread has been identified as through the foramen ovale [20,21]. Intracranial spread here appears to extend along the mandibular nerve, following tumor extension from the nasopharynx into the PPS (Fig. 6.7). This explains why intracranial spread often involves the gasserian ganglion. In some patients, tumor may be observed to extend further along the trigeminal nerve into the pons [22]. Involvement of the mandibular nerve often results in denervation atrophy of the muscles of mastication.

All the above paths of spread can lead to infiltration of the cavernous sinus, placing cranial nerves III, IV, the ophthalmic division of V and VI at risk. When tumor spreads posterolaterally into the jugular foramen and posterior cranial fossa, palsies of cranial nerves IX, X and XI may become evident.

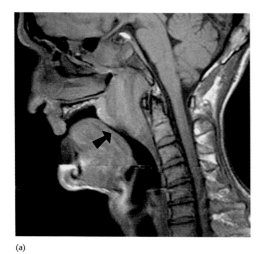
(a)

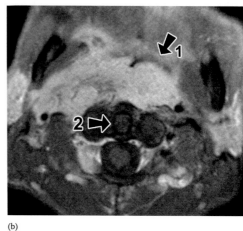
(b)

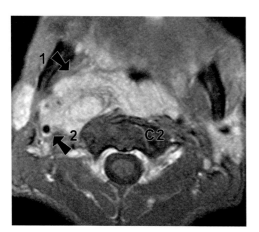
(c)

Fig. 6.6. Nasopharyngeal carcinoma with inferior spread. (a) Sagittal contrast-enhanced MRI shows tumor in the nasopharynx with inferior extension into the oropharynx (arrow). (b) Axial contrast-enhanced MRI shows a large tumor in the nasopharynx (arrow 1). Note that the dens is still visible (arrow 2). (c) Axial contrast-enhanced MRI shows nasopharyngeal carcinoma at the level of C2. The C1/C2 junction is used to demarcate the oropharynx from the nasopharynx. Note infiltration of right parapharyngeal and masticator spaces (arrow 1) and displacement of carotid sheath (arrow 2).

Volume of nasopharyngeal carcinomas

Tumor volume is now known to be a significant prognostic factor in the treatment of malignant tumors [23,24] and has also been reported for the treatment outcome of NPC [25–28]. Investigators have suggested the importance of incorporating tumor volume into the TNM staging system.

The probability of cure depends on a number of factors, including the initial number of tumor clonogens. It is also known that the number of tumor clonogens increases linearly with tumor volume. Hence, tumor volume can be a useful predictor (prognostic factor) of local treatment outcome [29]. If tumor prognosis

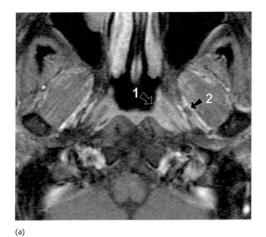

(a)

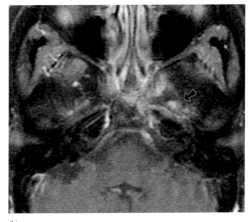

(b)

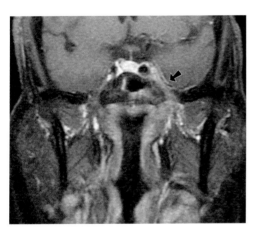

(c)

Fig. 6.7. Nasopharyngeal carcinoma with superior spread. (a) Axial contrast-enhanced MRI shows a small left tumor (arrow 1). Note the mandibular nerve in the parapharyngeal space (arrow 2). (b) Axial contrast-enhanced MRI (further superiorly) shows perineural spread involving the left mandibular nerve (arrow). (c) Coronal contrast-enhanced MRI shows intracranial spread through the left foramen ovale. Note the enlarged cavernous sinus (arrow).

depends on the number of tumor clonogens to be sterilized, it can be seen that a single dimensional measurement appears inadequate for prognostication. Hence a small tumor affecting a critical area may have a higher T classification compared with a large tumor confined to a defined anatomic site. Early investigations have demonstrated a positive relationship between NPC tumor volume and the TNM classification system [30].

If tumor volume is to be used as an independent prognostic factor, it is imperative that the methods for volume measurement be standardized, robust and reliable. Even today, technical considerations have prevented tumor-volume measurement from being routinely used in a clinical setting. The measurement of tumor volume has always been tedious. It involves tracing the tumor outline and then deriving the volume by summation of area techniques. Whether this process is carried out by a radiologist or by a technician, there is always an important element of subjectivity that results in both intra- and interoperator variation [31–33]. To overcome this problem, several investigators have developed semi-automated or automated systems to reduce both intra- and interoperator variability [34–36]. Errors encountered by computer-based techniques are then likely to be classified as systematic errors and not a result, for example, of the experience of the operator. Semi-automated tumor volume measurement is now possible for NPC [37].

Metastasis

Cervical lymphadenopathy is common in NPC. Often, it is the enlarged neck nodes that prompt initial medical consultation and 75% of patients have enlarged cervical nodes at presentation [38]. Bilateral lymphadenopathy may be seen in up to 80% of patients. Nodal metastasis, as a rule, shows an orderly inferior spread and the affected nodes are larger in the upper neck than in the more inferiorly situated nodes [39]. Lymphadenopathy of the LRP nodes may be seen in 65% of patients with cervical lymphadenopathy. Although the LRP nodes are considered first echelon nodes, 35% of metastases bypass the LRP nodes to reach the internal jugular nodes directly [38].

There is a high frequency of distant metastasis with NPC compared with other tumors of the head and neck [40]. The frequency of distant spread varies between 5% and 41%, compared with 5–24% in other head and neck tumors. The most common site of metastasis is bone (20%), followed by lung (13%) and liver (9%) [41].

Post-treatment imaging

The aim of follow-up is to detect early recurrence, allowing timely institution of appropriate therapy and thereby improving the survival rate. Imaging is also required for assessing treatment complications.

Tumor recurrence

The mainstay of treatment is radiation therapy. Patients with NPC are followed clinically and tumor recurrence is usually detected by endoscopy [42]. Imaging is requested for the assessment of tumor extent followed by biopsy confirmation.

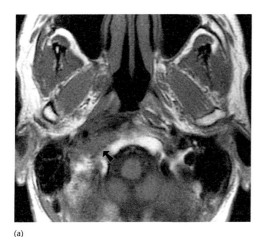
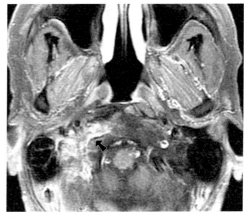

(a)   (b)

Fig. 6.8. Submucosal recurrence of nasopharyngeal carcinoma detected on imaging follow-up. (a) Axial T$_1$-weighted MRI shows an area of intermediate signal intensity (arrow) involving the prevertebral space. (b) Axial contrast-enhanced MRI shows heterogeneous tumor enhancement (arrow).

Imaging is also used to confirm deep recurrences not apparent on endoscopy but suspected on the basis of history and symptomology of routine imaging follow-up (Fig. 6.8). Following radiation therapy, excessive crust formation and mucosal bleeding often hampers endoscopy. These changes may last for years. Furthermore, the endoscopist may not detect submucosal recurrence. Imaging is particularly important in this group of patients.

Differentiating fibrosis from tumor recurrence is difficult using CT since the attenuation values of these tissues are similar. Separating tumor recurrence from fibrosis is only easier with MRI if the scar is mature. Early fibrous tissue is hypercellular and produces high signal intensity on T$_2$-weighted images. Both immature scar and tumor show contrast-enhancement on MRI and high signal intensity on T$_2$-weighted images. Mature scar, which is hypocellular, does not show contrast enhancement and is characterized by low signal intensity on T$_2$-weighted images.

The simultaneous dynamic processes of fibrosis and tissue reaction to irradiation often produce a confusing picture. Residual disease or recurrent tumor may be hypointense on T$_2$-weighted images relative to granulation tissue in the early stage. Scar tissue may also show high signal intensity in T$_2$-weighted images. Furthermore, areas of high signal intensity on T$_2$-weighted images may be seen in corresponding areas showing no contrast enhancement. Differentiating tumor recurrence from fibrosis can, therefore, be a formidable task [42].

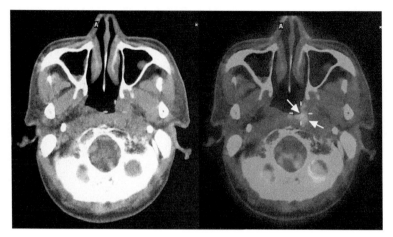

Fig. 6.9. Recurrence of nasopharyngeal carcinoma demonstrated by PET–CT. Axial CT showed no mass lesion in the left fossa of Rosenmuller but a fused PET–CT image demonstrates tracer uptake (arrows).

It is important to obtain a baseline study around 3 to 6 months after radiation therapy, which can be used for comparison in future studies. It is often very helpful to compare suspected recurrence with previous examinations. A stable appearance can provide reassurance that the abnormality seen is most likely to be caused by post-radiation change. In the first year, a 6-monthly examination will provide early information regarding persistent tumor or early recurrence. Subsequent imaging follow-up is recommended on a yearly basis for 3 years, after which clinical follow-up will suffice. Most relapses will occur within 3 years following treatment.

Positron emission tomography (PET) using ^{18}F-fluorodeoxyglucose has demonstrated value in detecting NPC recurrence following radiotherapy (Fig. 6.9). The advent of PET–CT has provided even more information by co-registering tracer uptake with anatomical information.

Complications of therapy

The complications of radiation therapy can be divided into neurological and non-neurological sequelae. Neurological complications include temporal lobe necrosis, (TLN), encephalomyelopathy and cranial nerve palsies. Non-neurological complications include atrophy of salivary glands and the muscles of mastication and otological deficiencies.

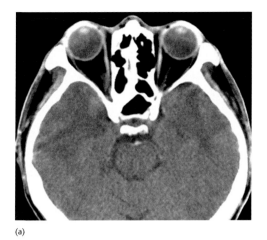

(a)

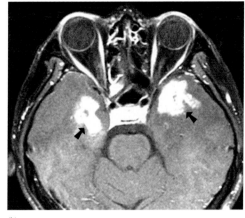

(b)

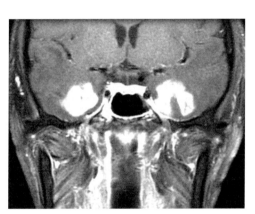

(c)

Fig. 6.10. Temporal lobe necrosis. (a) Axial contrast-enhanced CT shows bilateral heterogeneous low-attenuation lesions in the temporal lobes. (b) Axial contrast-enhanced MRI shows enhancing lesions (arrows) in the temporal lobes, with perilesional edema. (c) Coronal contrast-enhanced MRI shows enhancing lesions in the inferomedial aspect of both temporal lobes.

Neurological complications

During radiation therapy, the inferior and medial portions of both temporal lobes are often included in the target volume. This becomes inevitable when tumor extension into the intracranial cavity is demonstrated. The cumulative incidence of TLN is 3% [43,44]. The latent interval ranges from 1.5 to 13 years (median, 5 years). The occurrence of TLN is probably under diagnosed, as 39% of patients have only vague symptoms while 16% have none at all. The risk of TLN is also related to dose and fractionation. Hypofraction radiation therapy techniques increase the risk of brain damage [45–47].

Cerebral edema is the earliest radiological sign. This is followed by foci of necrosis, which may be located in the gray matter, white matter or both (Fig. 6.10). White matter lesions are characteristically associated with florid edema [48]. Lesions in the gray matter may have minimal or no edema. Although cerebral edema is generally considered an acute to subacute sign of injury, in TLN this sign often persists for years [48]. Early lesions may heal completely but extensive lesions frequently show temporal lobe atrophy or macrocystic encephalomalacia.

The most important differential diagnosis of TLN is tumor recurrence. An important point of distinction is whereas recurrent skull base tumor is an extra-axial lesion, TLN is an intra-axial pathological process. In addition, NPC with intracranial extension, unlike TLN, is usually not associated with cerebral edema. Magnetic resonance spectroscopy may be used to separate TLN from tumor recurrence with brain invasion. It is important to note that skull base tumors are not expected to show N-acetyl-aspartate (NAA) since this is a neuronal marker. In the early delayed phase of TLN, the levels of N-acetyl-aspartate and creatine are reduced, but choline may be raised, thus mimicking a primary brain tumor. The increased choline is the result of demyelination secondary to injury to oligodendrocytes. The late delayed phase of radiation injury shows the decrease of N-acetyl-aspartate, choline and creatine [49]. However, PET–CT often provides an easier, though more expensive, method of differentiating tumor recurrence from TLN. Typically, recurrent tumors show uptake of radionuclide tracer while necrotic brain tissue does not.

Radiation-associated tumors

The carcinogenic potential of ionizing radiation is a well-recognized but poorly understood phenomenon. The term radiation-induced tumors is frequently used to describe second tumors within previously irradiated fields. However, ascribing the second tumor as a direct product of irradiation is often difficult. This entity is better called radiation-associated tumors.

The criteria for diagnosing such tumors include (a) history of radiation therapy, (b) the second neoplasm must occur within the field of radiation, (c) the histology of the second neoplasm must be distinctly different from the primary tumor, and (d) a latency period, arbitrarily of at least 5 years between radiation therapy and the occurrence of the second tumor [50].

The frequency of radiation-associated tumors of the head and neck is unknown, although it has been estimated to be between 0.4% and 0.7% [51,52]. Depending on the initial site of radiation, the types of tumor reported include sarcomas, meningiomas, schwannomas, gliomas and thyroid tumors [53,54]. Malignancies following radiation therapy for NPC have also been reported, including sarcomas and squamous cell carcinomas in the temporal bone [55–57]. The improvement of radiation therapy techniques has contributed to increased survival rates for patients with NPC. We can, therefore, expect to see more long-term complications such as radiation-associated tumors.

Bone changes

Osteoradionecrosis, which is believed to be secondary to osteoblastic destruction with subsequent vascular damage, may occur approximately 1 year after irradiation and is slowly progressive [58]. In the treatment of NPC, the bones most frequently involved include the skull base and the mandible.

Imaging findings include areas of osteolysis and mixed sclerosis within the irradiation portal. Deep gas-containing ulcerations, sclerosis, fragmentation and sloughing of necrotic bone as well as surrounding inflammatory soft tissue swelling may also be seen [59]. The imaging appearance of osteoradionecrosis may mimic tumor recurrence or osteomyelitis. The absence of an associated soft tissue mass with osteoradionecrosis may be helpful in differentiating between these two entities. However, osteonecrosis with superimposed infection is quite common. Sometimes, osteoradionecrosis can be associated with prominent soft-tissue thickening and enhancement in the adjacent musculature [60]. When a bulky soft tissue mass is seen in conjunction with osteoradionecrosis, a biopsy should be performed to exclude tumor recurrence.

Conclusions

The nasopharynx is located just below the central skull base and neoplasms in this region are relatively inaccessible to physical examination. Although endoscopy provides useful information on mucosal involvement, it cannot delineate the full extent of the submucosal, osseous or intracranial components of the disease. Hence, clinical staging, assessment of tumor recurrence and treatment complications are largely dependent on imaging. Familiarity with the complex anatomy of the nasopharynx, the natural history of NPC and post-treatment findings facilitates the accurate mapping of tumor extent and the identification of post-radiation therapy complications.

REFERENCES

1. International Agency for Research on Cancer. *Cancer Incidence in Five Continents*, vol. VII. (*Scientific Publication* No. 143, ed. D. M. Parkin, S. L. Whelan, J. Ferlay, *et al.*) (Lyon: IRAC Press, 1997).
2. P. H. K. Choi, M. W. M. Sven, D. P. Huang, *et al.* Nasopharyngeal carcinoma: genetic changes, Epstein–Barr virus infection, or both. A clinical and molecular study of 36 patients. *Cancer* **72** (1993), 2873–2878.
3. J. H. C. Ho. An epidemiologic and clinical study of nasopharyngeal carcinoma. *Int J Radiat Oncol Biol Phys* **4** (1978), 182–198.

4. V. F. H. Chong, Y. F. Fan. Radiology of the masticator space. *Clin Radiol* **51** (1996), 457–465.

5. M. M. Hsu, Y. H. Young, K. L. Lin. Eustachian tube function of patients with nasopharyngeal carcinoma. *Ann Otol Rhinol Laryngol* **104** (1995), 453–455.

6. J. S. T. Sham, W. I. Wei, S. K. Lau, *et al.* Serous otitis media and paranasopharyngeal extension of nasopharyngeal carcinoma. *Head Neck* **14** (1992), 19–23.

7. J. S. T. Sham, Y. K. Cheung, D. Choy, *et al.* Nasopharyngeal carcinoma: CT evaluation of patterns of tumor spread. *Am J Neurolradiol* **12** (1991), 265–270.

8. V. F. H. Chong, Y. F. Fan. Nasopharyngeal carcinoma. *Semin Ultrasound CT MR* **19** (1998), 449–462.

9. F. L. Greene, D. L. Page, I. D. Fleming, *et al. AJCC Cancer Staging Manual*, 6th edn (New York: Springer-Verlag, 2002).

10. V. F. H. Chong, Y. F. Fan. Pterygopalatine fossa and maxillary nerve infiltration in nasopharyngeal carcinoma. *Head Neck* **19** (1997), 121–125.

11. V. F. H. Chong, Y. F. Fan. Pictorial essay: maxillary nerve involvement in nasopharyngeal carcinoma. *Am J Roentgenol* **167** (1996), 1309–1312.

12. V. F. H. Chong. Masticator space in nasopharyngeal carcinoma. *Ann Otol Rhinol Laryngol* **106** (1997), 979–982.

13. V. F. H. Chong, Y. F. Fan. Jugular foramen involvement in nasopharyngeal carcinoma. *J Laryngol Otol* **110** (1996), 897–900.

14. V. F. H. Chong, Y. F. Fan. Radiology of the carotid space. *Clin Radiol* **51** (1996), 762–768.

15. V. F. H. Chong, Y. F. Fan, J. B. K. Khoo. Nasopharyngeal carcinoma with intracranial spread: CT and MRI characteristics. *J Comput Assist Tomogr* **20** (1996), 563–639.

16. A. J. Silver, M. E. Mawad, S. K. Hilal, *et al.* Computed tomography of the nasopharynx and related spaces. Part 1: Anatomy. *Radiology* **147** (1993), 725–731.

17. H. M. Neel. Malignant neoplasm of the nasopharynx. In *Otolaryngology: Head and Neck Surgery*, vol. 2, ed. D. E. Schuller (St. Louis: Mosby, 1986), pp. 1401–1411.

18. H. D. Curtin, W. L. Hirsch. Base of the skull. In *Magnetic Resonance Imaging of the Brain and Spine*, ed. S. W. Atlas (New York: Raven Press, 1991), pp. 669–707.

19. J. S. T. Sham, Y. K. Cheung, D. Choy, *et al.* Cranial nerve involvement and base of skull erosion in nasopharyngeal carcinoma. *Cancer* **68** (1991), 422–426.

20. V. F. H. Chong, Y. F. Fan, J. B. K. Khoo. Nasopharyngeal carcinoma with intracranial spread: CT and MRI characteristics. *J Comput Assist Tomogr* **20** (1996), 563–639.

21. C. Y. Su, C. C. Lui. Perineural invasion of the trigeminal nerve in patients with nasopharyngeal carcinoma. *Cancer* **78** (1996), 2063–2069.

22. V. F. H. Chong. Trigeminal neuralgia in nasopharyngeal carcinoma. *J Laryngol Otol* **110** (1996), 394–396.

23. D. J. Brenner. Dose, volume and tumor control predictions in radiotherapy. *Int J Radiat Oncol Biol Phys* **26** (1993), 171–179.

24. C. R. Johnson, H. D. Thames, D. T. Huang, *et al*. The tumor volume and clonogen number relationship: tumor control predictions based upon tumor volume estimates derived from computed tomography. *Int J Radiat Oncol Biol Phys* **33** (1995), 281–287.

25. D. T. Chua, J. S. Sham, D. L. Kwong, *et al*. Volumetric analysis of tumor extent in nasopharyngeal carcinoma and correlation with treatment outcome. *Int J Radiat Oncol Biol Phys* **39** (1997), 711–719.

26. J. Willner, K. Baier, L. Pfreunder, *et al*. Tumor volume and local control in primary radiotherapy of nasopharyngeal carcinoma. *Acta Oncol* **38** (1999), 1025–1030.

27. M. K. Chen, T. H. Chen, J. P. Liu, *et al*. Better prediction of prognosis for patients with nasopharyngeal carcinoma using primary tumor volume. *Cancer* **100** (2004), 2160–2166.

28. W. M. Sze, A. W. M. Lee, T. K. Yau, *et al*. Primary tumor volume of nasopharyngeal carcinoma: prognostic significance of local control. *Int J Radiat Oncol Biol Phys* **59** (2004), 21–27.

29. R. Hermans. Head and neck cancer: how imaging predicts treatment outcome. *Cancer Imaging* **6** (2006), S145–S153.

30. V. F. H. Chong, J. Y. Zhou, J. B. K. Khoo, K. L. Chan, J. Huang. Correlation between MR imaging-derived nasopharyngeal carcinoma tumor-volume and TNM System. *Int J Radiat Oncol Biol Phys* **64** (2006), 72–76.

31. L. P. Clarke, R. P. Velthuizen, M. A. Camacho, *et al*. MRI segmentation: methods and applications. *Magn Reson Imaging* **13** (1995), 343–368.

32. E. J. Zijlstra, M. J. Taphoorn, F. Barkhof, *et al*. Radiotherapy response of cerebral metastases quantified by serial MR imaging. *J Neurooncol* **21** (1994), 171–176.

33. R. K. Ten Haken, A. F. Thorton Jr., H. M. Sandler, *et al*. A quantitative assessment of the addition of MRI to CT-based, 3-D treatment planning of brain tumors. *Radiother Oncol* **25** (1992), 121–133.

34. L. R. Schad, S. Blum, I. Zuna. MR tissue characterization of intracranial tumors by means of textual analysis. *Magn Reson Imaging* **11** (1993), 889–896.

35. R. P. Velthuizen, L. P. Clark, S. Phuphanich, *et al*. Unsupervised measurement of brain tumor volume on MR images. *J Magn Reson Imaging* **5** (1995), 594–605.

36. W. E. Phillips, R. P. Velthuizen, S. Phuphanich, *et al*. Applications of fuzzy c-means segmentation technique for tissue differentiation in MR images of hemorrhagic glioblastoma multiforme. *Magn Reson Imaging* **13** (1995), 277–290.

37. V. F. H. Chong, J. Y. Zhou, J. B. K. Khoo, J. Huang, T. K. Lim. Tumor volume measurement in nasopharyngeal carcinoma. *Radiology* **231** (2004), 914–921.

38. V. F. H. Chong, Y. F. Fan, J. B. K. Khoo. Retropharyngeal lymphadenopathy in nasopharyngeal carcinoma. *Eur J Radiol* **21** (1995), 100–105.

39. J. S. T. Sham, D. Choy, W. I. Wei. Nasopharyngeal carcinoma: orderly neck node spread. *Int J Radiat Oncol Biol Phys* **19** (1990), 929–933.

40. O. R. Merino, R. D. Linberg, G. H. Fletcher. An analysis of distant metastases from squamous cell carcinoma of the upper respiratory and digestive tracts. *Cancer* **40** (1977), 145–51.

41. J. S. T. Sham, Y. K. Cheung, F. L. Chan, *et al.* Nasopharyngeal carcinoma: pattern of skeletal metastases. *Br J Radiol* **63** (1990), 202–205.

42. V. F. H. Chong, Y. F. Fan. Detection of recurrent nasopharyngeal carcinoma: CT vs MR imaging. *Radiology* **202** (1997), 453–470.

43. A. W. M. Lee, S. C. K. Law, S. H. Ng, *et al.* Retrospective analysis of nasopharyngeal carcinoma treated during 1976–1985: late complications following megavoltage irradiation. *Br J Radiol* **65** (1992), 918–928.

44. A. W. N. Lee, S. H. Ng, J. H. C. Ho, *et al.* Clinical diagnosis of late temporal lobe necrosis following radiation therapy for nasopharyngeal carcinoma. *Cancer* **61** (1988), 1535–1542.

45. A. W. M. Lee, W. Foo, R. Chappell, *et al.* Effect of time, dose, and fractionation on temporal lobe necrosis following radiotherapy for nasopharyngeal carcinoma. *Int J Radiat Oncol Biol Phys* **40** (1998), 35–42.

46. Y. M. Jen, W. L. Hsu, C. Y. Chen, *et al.* Different risks of symptomatic brain necrosis in NPC patients treated with different altered fractionated radiotherapy techniques. *Int J Radiat Oncol Biol Phys* **51** (2001), 344–348.

47. A. W. M. Lee, D. L. Kwong, S. F. Leung, *et al.* Factors affecting risk of symptomatic temporal lobe necrosis: significance of fractional dose and treatment time. *Int J Radiat Oncol Biol Phys* **53** (2002), 75–85.

48. V. F. H. Chong, Y. F. Fan, Y. F. Mukherji. Radiation-induced temporal lobe changes: CT and MR imaging characteristics. *Am J Radiol* **175** (2000), 431–436.

49. V. F. H. Chong, H. Rumpel, Y. S. Aw, *et al.* Temporal lobe necrosis following radiation therapy for nasopharyngeal carcinoma: proton MR spectroscopic findings. *Int J Radiat Oncol Biol Phys* **45** (1999), 699–705.

50. W. G. Cahan, H. G. Woodward, N. L. Higinbotham, Stewart F. W. L. Coley sarcoma arising in irradiated bone: report of eleven cases. *Cancer* **1** (1948), 3–29.

51. R. A. Steeves, J. P. Bataini. Neoplasms induced by megavoltage radiation in the head and neck region. *Cancer* **47** (1981), 1770–1774.

52. B. F. van der Laan, G. Baris, R. T. Gregor, F. J. Hilgers, A. J. Balm. Radiation-induced tumors of the head and neck. *J Laryngol Otol* **109** (1995), 346–349.

53. R. J. Mark, J. W. Bailet, J. Poen, *et al.* Post-radiation sarcoma of the head and neck. *Cancer* **72** (1993), 887–893.

54. A. B. Rubinstein, E. Reichenthal, H. Borohov. Radiation-induced schwannomas. *Neurosurgery* **24** (1989), 929–932.

55. Y. H. Goh, V. F. H. Chong, W. K. Low. Temporal bone tumors in patients irradiated for nasopharyngeal neoplasms. *J Laryngol Otol* **113** (1999), 222–228.

56. L. H. Y. Lim, Y. H. Goh, Y. M. Chan, V. F. H. Chong, W. K. Low. Malignancy of the temporal bone and external auditory canal. *Otolaryngol Head Neck Surg* **122** (2000), 882–886.

57. A. D. King, A. T. Ahuja, P. M. Teo, *et al.* Radiation induced sarcomas of the head and neck following radiotherapy for nasopharyngeal carcinoma. *Clin Radiol* **55** (2000), 684–689.

58. K. Shimanovskaya, A. Shimen. *Radiation Injury of Bone.* (New York: Pergamon, 1983), pp. 57–83.

59. M. Becker, G. Schroth, P. Zbaren. Long-term changes induced by high-dose irradiation of the head and neck region: imaging findings. *RadioGraphics* **17** (1997), 5–26.

60. J. Chong, L. K. Hinckley, L. E. Ginsberg. Masticator space abnormalities associated with mandibular osteoradionecrosis: MR and CT findings in five patients. *Am J Neuroradiol* **21** (2000), 175–178.

7

Neck and distant disease spread

Ann D. King

Nodal metastases

Background

Cervical nodal metastases have a significant impact on the outcome of patients with squamous cell cancer (SCC) of the head and neck (HNSCC). Nodal metastases are a cause of mortality in patients in whom the primary cancer is controlled, and they increase the risk of distant metastases. Prognosis decreases with increasing nodal stage and overall the rate of cure is halved in those patients with nodal spread. Classification of nodal groups was based originally on anatomical location according to Rouvière [1] and later adapted to surgical levels [2,3]. These surgical levels have since been translated to radiological levels using anatomical landmarks on axial computed tomography (CT) [4] and are in the process of being adapted to clinical target volumes for image-guided radiotherapy [5]. Both anatomical sites and levels are currently used in clinical practice (Fig. 7.1). Disease within the nodes tends to spread in an orderly fashion down the neck, although skip metastases are found in 5% of patients and routes of spread may be altered by bulky nodal disease and previous treatment. The sites of preferential nodal spread from primary HNSCC are shown in Table 7.1. Staging nodal metastases is performed using the TNM classification set out by the American Joint Committee on Cancer [6] (Table 7.2). For nodal staging purposes, 3 and 6 cm are the important size criteria. Nodal metastases denote advanced stage disease (N1, stage III; N2, stage IV). This classification is applied to nodes from all primary sites of HNSCC with the exception of nodes from nasopharyngeal carcinoma (see footnote to Table 7.2).

Morphological imaging of nodal metastases

Criteria for diagnosis of a metastatic node

The morphological modalities of CT, magnetic resonance imaging (MRI) and ultrasound are employed most commonly to detect metastatic nodes. The identification of

Squamous Cell Cancer of the Neck, ed. Robert Hermans. Published by Cambridge University Press.

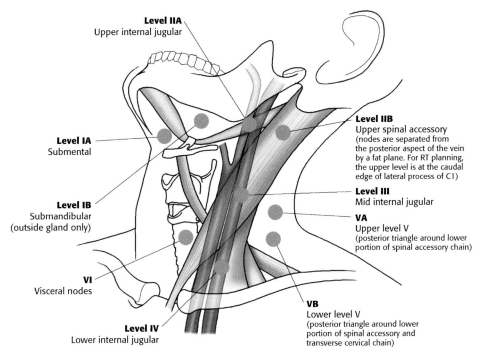

Level IIA
Upper internal jugular

Level IIB
Upper spinal accessory
(nodes are separated from
the posterior aspect of the vein
by a fat plane. For RT planning,
the upper level is at the caudal
edge of lateral process of C1)

Level IA
Submental

Level IB
Submandibular
(outside gland only)

Level III
Mid internal jugular

VA
Upper level V
(posterior triangle around lower
portion of spinal accessory chain)

VI
Visceral nodes

VB
Lower level V
(posterior triangle around lower
portion of spinal accessory and
transverse cervical chain)

Level IV
Lower internal jugular

Fig. 7.1. Nodal groups in the neck according to anatomical sites and surgical levels. Additional nodal groups according to site are (1) the facial, parotid, auricular and suboccipital nodes, (2) the retropharyngeal nodes, (3) the supraclavicular nodes, and (4) the superior mediastinal nodes (level VII in some surgical classification systems). Color version in plate section.

a malignant node depends upon the criteria of (1) size, (2) shape, (3) internal architecture and (4) image-guided biopsy.

Size

The maximum size of the minimum diameter is used to identify an enlarged node (as opposed to the maximum size of the maximum diameter, which is used for staging purposes; see Table 7.2). Unfortunately, some enlarged nodes are reactive while some non-enlarged nodes harbor metastatic deposits. In general, the smaller the cut-off threshold for a node the higher the sensitivity and lower the specificity for detection of malignancy. This point is well illustrated by Curtin *et al.* [7], who showed that the sensitivity for detection of metastatic nodes by CT decreased from 98% to 56% and the specificity increased from 13% to 84% when the threshold for size was changed from 5 to 15 mm. In addition, there are many factors that influence the size of normal nodes. These include previous treatment, patient age and nodal site (nodes

Table 7.1. Primary cancers: paths of spread of nodal metastases

Site of primary cancer	Nodal groups	Comments
Nasopharynx	Retropharyngeal nodes and upper internal jugular/spinal accessory nodes (level IIA, B), then down the neck	Bilateral (including retropharyngeal nodes) in 60%
Oral cavity (oral tongue and floor of mouth)	Submental (IA) and submandibular (IB) nodes, but lateral part of tongue and more posterior floor of mouth drain to the upper internal jugular (IIA) and then upper spinal accessory (IIB) nodes	Metastases from the lateral margin of the oral tongue may go directly to level IV
Oropharynx (tongue base, palatine tonsil and soft palate)	Upper internal jugular and spinal accessory (IIA, B) and sometimes submandibular (IB) nodes; also may directly spread to mid internal jugular (III) and retropharyngeal nodes	Contralateral nodes in 20% of tumors in the base of the tongue and soft palate
Hypopharynx	Mid (III) and lower (IV) internal jugular and sometimes upper internal jugular/spinal accessory (IIA, B) nodes; posterior wall tumors spread to the retropharyngeal nodes	Increased risk of contralateral node involvement if the tumor crosses the midline or involves the medial wall of the pyriform sinus
Larynx	Supraglottis and glottis to upper internal jugular and spinal accessory nodes (IIA, B) and to mid internal jugular nodes (III); subglottis to mid (III) and lower (IV) internal jugular nodes	Supraglottis and subglottis have a rich lymphatic supply so incidence of node involvement is high compared with the low incidence (0–10% in T1 and T2) from tumors of the glottis, which has a poor lymphatic supply
Skin	Dependent on site of the tumor but often involves superficial nodal groups such as the periauricular, parotid and facial	

Table 7.2. Nodal staging of head and neck squamous cell carcinoma (with exception of nasopharyngeal carcinoma^a) according to the 6th edition of the American Joint Committee on Cancer classification (2002)

Regional lymph nodes (N)	Description
NX	Regional lymph nodes cannot be assessed
N0	No regional lymph node metastasis
N1	Metastasis in a single ipsilateral lymph node, $\leqslant 3$ cm in greatest dimension
N2	Metastasis in a single ipsilateral node, > 3 cm and $\leqslant 6$ cm in greatest dimension; or in multiple ipsilateral lymph nodes, $\leqslant 6$ cm in greatest dimension; or in bilateral or contralateral lymph nodes, $\leqslant 6$ cm in greatest dimension
N2a	Metastasis in single ipsilateral lymph node > 3 cm and $\leqslant 6$ cm in greatest dimension
N2b	Metastasis in multiple ipsilateral lymph nodes $\leqslant 6$ cm in greatest dimension
N2c	Metastasis in bilateral or contralateral lymph nodes, $\leqslant 6$ cm in greatest dimension
N3	Metastasis in a lymph node > 6 cm in greatest dimension

^{a} For nasopharyngeal carcinoma, nodes in the supraclavicular fossa are an ominous sign and this is reflected in the staging system, N3 nodes are either > 6 cm or extend to supraclavicular fossa, all other nodes are classified as N1 if unilateral and N2 if bilateral (N1 signifies stage IIB, N2 stage III, N3 stage IV).
From Greene *et al.* (2002) [6].

are small in the retropharyngeal region below the skull base, peak in size in the jugulodigastric region and then gradually decrease in size again on descending the neck). In 1990, van den Brekel *et al.* [8] proposed using a cut-off value of 11 mm at level II and 10 mm for nodes elsewhere, together with grouping of three or more nodes of 8–10 mm in size. These are still the most widely used criteria today for assessing nodal size, although in order to improve sensitivity, thresholds of 7 mm at level II and 6 mm in the rest of the neck have been proposed [9].

Shape
Normal nodes are oval in shape while malignant nodes become round. This assessment tends to be made on visual inspection but can be quantified by

measuring the ratio of the long to the short axis; a ratio of < 2 has been reported to have an accuracy of 95% for detecting metastatic nodes [10].

Internal architecture

Ultrasound, CT and MRI present similar problems when using the criteria of size and shape and so the relative strengths and weaknesses of each modality depend on the ability to identify abnormalities of internal architecture.

Necrosis. In populations where the prevalence of infection is low, necrosis is one of the most accurate signs of a metastatic node. Necrosis is common in metastatic nodes from SCC, being found in 50% of nodes > 1.5 cm in size and 10–33% of nodes of ≤ 1 cm. Necrosis on CT, MRI and ultrasound is demonstrated in Fig. 7.2. All three techniques have difficulty in detecting necrosis that is < 3 mm in size. Above 3 mm in size, both CT and MRI have a similar sensitivity (91–93%), while the sensitivity is lower for ultrasound (77%) because small foci of isoechoic necrosis may be missed [11] (Fig. 7.2d). The specificity of all three techniques is similar (90%) with small tumor and keratin deposits from SCC giving a similar appearance to necrosis.

Extranodal neoplastic spread (ENS). This is associated with an increase in locoregional recurrence, distant metastases and decreased survival. In the absence of infection or previous treatment, ENS is an accurate sign of a metastatic node. Extranodal spread is seen as an irregular nodal border, nodular capsular enhancement and infiltration into adjacent tissues (Fig. 7.2b). As nodes increase in size, the incidence of ENS increases, so that ENS is found in 25% of nodes measuring 1 cm, 50% measuring 2–3 cm and 75% measuring > 3 cm. Spread occurs also in nodes as small as 5 mm, and the detection of ENS in these non-enlarged nodes has the potential to improve diagnostic accuracy of imaging. Extranodal spread is detected by MRI and CT with similar accuracy [12], while the accuracy of ultrasound is unknown. Imaging detection of ENS into adjacent structures is important for planning surgical resection and for those patients undergoing chemoradiotherapy. It is the only method to detect this important prognostic sign.

Hilum architecture. The nodal hilum is made up of lymphatic sinuses and vessels, and with age it may become more prominent through fatty deposition. For practical purposes, normal and reactive nodes have a hilum while metastatic nodes lose the hilum. The normal hilum is not identified consistently by CT or MRI but ultrasound is able to identify the normal hilum in 90% of nodes < 5 mm [13] (Fig. 7.3a); this figure increases to 99% when Doppler is used to show the hilar vascularity. The loss of hilum can be seen by ultrasound in > 90% of metastatic nodes [14] (Fig. 7.3b).

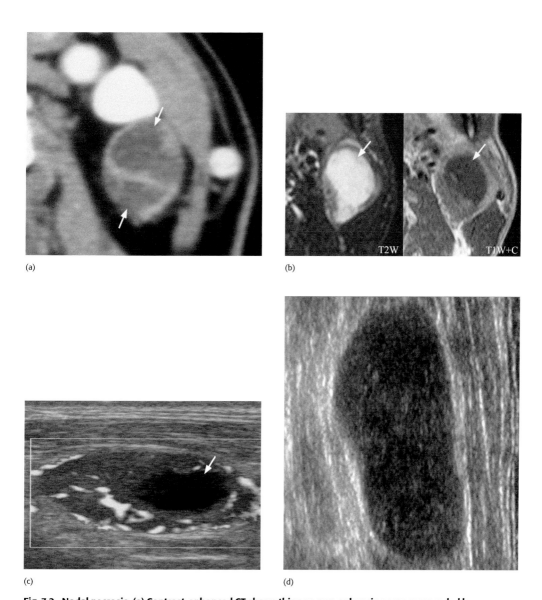

Fig. 7.2. Nodal necrosis. (a) Contrast-enhanced CT shows this as a non-enhancing area surrounded by an enhancing rim of residual nodal tissue (arrows). (b) On MRI it appears as an area of very high signal intensity on T_2-weighted images and low signal intensity with an enhancing rim of residual nodal tissue on contrast-enhanced T_1-weighted images (this node also shows early extranodal neoplasmic spread). (c,d) On ultrasound nodal necrosis appears as an avascular area of low echogenicity (c), but it can be isoechoic on ultrasound and therefore difficult to detect (d, same node as illustrated in [a]). (Part (c) is available in color in the plate section.)

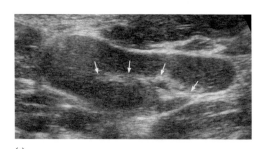
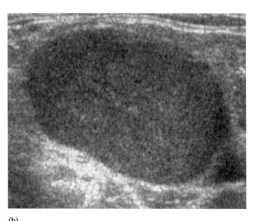

(a)   (b)

Fig. 7.3. Ultrasound of lymph node. (a) A normal oval-shaped node with a hilum (arrows) consisting of vessels, lymphatic sinuses and a variable amount of fat. (b) Loss of the hilum in a metastatic node in squamous cell carcinoma.

Vascularity.   Detection of vascularity is one of the major advantages of color Doppler ultrasound. Normal nodes have a hilar vascular pattern (Fig. 7.4a), which is seen as vascularity at the hilum that fans out to the periphery. Malignant nodes develop an abnormal peripheral pattern of vessels, with infiltration of vessels into the node from the periphery (Fig. 7.4b) [15] while the hilar pattern of vascularity may be either retained or lost.

Calcification.   Nodal calcification is extremely rare in SCC and its presence suggests other diagnoses, most notably nodes affected by papillary carcinoma of the thyroid.

Image-guided biopsy
Image-guided biopsy is best achieved using the real-time guidance of ultrasound, and in experienced hands nodes as small as 4–5 mm may be successfully diagnosed using fine-needle aspiration cytology (FNAC) [16].

Strategy for imaging and impact on management
It is difficult to compare the accuracy of CT, MRI and ultrasound because there is great variability in the reported results [17]. This is not surprising given that there is great variability in (a) the scanning technique within each modality, (b) the criteria for diagnosis of a metastatic node within each modality and between modalities, (c) the patient population (N+ or N0 groups), and (d) the radiological–pathological

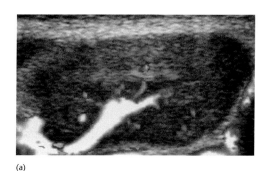
(a)

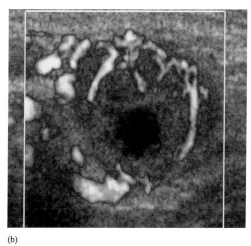
(b)

Fig. 7.4. Color Doppler ultrasound of a lymph node. (a) A normal node showing the hilar vascular pattern. (b) A necrotic metastatic node showing a peripheral vascular pattern. Color version in plate section.

correlation (FNAC versus fine serial sectioning). However, from the above discussion, it can be seen that ultrasound has several advantages over CT and MRI, namely identification of the nodal hilum, vascularity and image-guided biopsy. Van den Brekel *et al.* [18] reported a higher accuracy for ultrasound-guided FNAC (93%) than ultrasound alone (75%), CT (78%) or MRI (82%). Three other reported series have shown the advantages of ultrasound or ultrasound-guided biopsy over CT/MRI [19–21]. Currently, no imaging technique is able to detect micrometastases (defined as nodal deposits of < 2 or < 3 mm).

The modality of choice for imaging HNSCC is dictated by the primary rather than the nodal disease, so it usually lies between MRI or CT. With the exception of retropharyngeal nodes, which are better demonstrated by MRI, these two modalities have a similar performance in detecting metastatic nodes. Ultrasound is used to evaluate nodes in patients with early T stage disease where MRI/CT is not deemed necessary to evaluate the primary tumor. Ultrasound can be used also as an additional examination to MRI/CT when its advantages are likely to have an important impact on patient management.

In order to understand the possible impact of ultrasound, one has to understand current treatment options for nodal metastases. Surgery has been the mainstay of treatment for HNSCC nodal metastases. The surgical approach to the N0 neck is to remove sites of likely occult metastases using either a selective neck dissection (performed for staging purposes), or a modified radical neck dissection (aimed at curative intent). A "wait and see" approach may be taken if the perceived risk of occult metastases is judged to be < 20% [22], which, in practice, tends to be patients with small T1 tumors at sites in the oral cavity and glottis. The surgical approach to the N+ neck involves a radical neck dissection or a modified radical neck dissection. Currently, there is some evidence to suggest that the prognosis of patients with a single node (< 3 cm and no ENS) is similar to that of patients with no nodes, and so a possible role for a selective neck dissection is proposed for this group of N+ patients with limited disease [23]. Ultrasound has the greatest impact in patients with an N0 neck or a few borderline enlarged nodes on MRI/CT. Ultrasound confirmation of an N0 neck or an early N+ neck improves the clinician's confidence that the appropriate therapy is being initiated. For the "wait and see" approach, ultrasound also forms a vital part of follow-up, which involves frequent ultrasound examinations every 8–12 weeks [24]. Finding a small metastatic node in the N0 neck will convert the patient to a more aggressive approach, and vice versa if borderline nodes are found to be reactive rather than malignant. The impact of ultrasound on surgery planning is less for patients with multiple nodes because these patients will undergo a radical neck dissection or a modified version, although it must be remembered that both sides of the neck need to be considered separately. Recently, the role of chemoradiotherapy has been expanding and it now rivals surgery as the treatment of choice for advanced stage III and IV HNSCC [25]. At present, ultrasound has less impact in planning chemoradiotherapy, but with the advent of intensity-modulated radiotherapy the role of ultrasound for identifying specific groups of abnormal nodes will increase.

Functional imaging of nodal metastases

Imaging HNSCC is shifting from the morphological techniques of ultrasound, MRI and CT to the functional techniques such as positron emission tomography (PET) with ^{18}F-Fluorodioxyglucose (FDG) and functional MRI. These techniques are able to assess different aspects of the cancer microenvironment. The potential role of these functional techniques to identify metastatic nodes and predict/monitor cancer response are discussed below, while the role of functional nodal imaging in the post-treatment neck will be discussed in Chapter 8.

Positron emission tomography
Nodal metastases from SCC are FDG PET avid. When compared with the morphological techniques FDG PET appears to perform as well as or slightly better than morphological imaging [26]. However, FDG PET produces both false-positive and

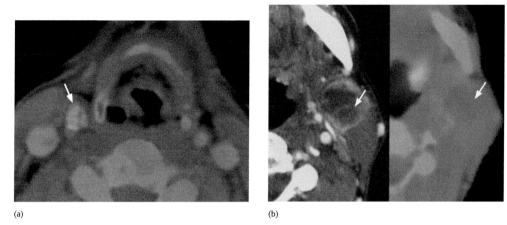

(a)   (b)

Fig. 7.5. Use of PET with ^{18}F-fluorodeoxyglucose (FDG). (a) A false-positive result where the right-sided node was reactive rather than metastatic on excision biopsy. (b) The necrotic portion of the left-sided metastastic node, shown on the T$_1$-weighted MRI post-contrast, fails to take up FDG (arrows); in a completely necrotic node this can lead to a false-negative result. Color version in plate section.

false-negative results. False-positive results arise most frequently from reactive nodes, which have standardized uptake values that overlap with malignant nodes [27] (Fig. 7.5a). Reactive nodes cause problems in clinical practice. When a node is identified as malignant by FDG PET alone, and this node has a major influence on treatment planning, the diagnosis may need to be confirmed by ultrasound-guided FNAC. False-negative results are found with small nodes, necrotic nodes (Fig. 7.5b) and where the node cannot be distinguished anatomically from the adjacent primary cancer. The predictive value of FDG uptake has been studied in relationship to the prediction of cancer treatment response, and while there are conflicting results, those cancers with a higher standardized uptake value tend to show less response [28].

Functional magnetic resonance imaging

Magnetic resonance is a versatile modality that can be used to assess different functional aspects of nodes. These include diffusion-weighted imaging (DWI), dynamic contrast-enhanced MRI (DCE-MRI), proton magnetic resonance spectroscopy (^{1}H-MRS) and ultrasmall super paramagnetic iron oxide particles.

Diffusion-weighted imaging

The mobility of water in different tissues can be measured to generate DWIs and apparent diffusion coefficient (ADC) maps. It is a quick technique that can be added to the conventional MRI examination. There are differences in the cellularity,

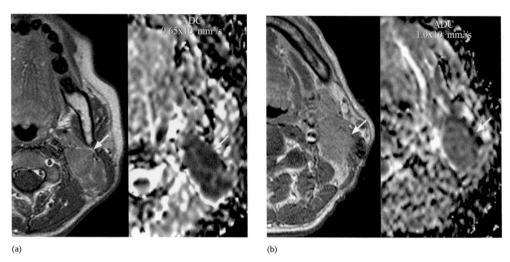

(a)   (b)

Fig. 7.6. Apparent diffusion coefficient (ADC) maps. (a) A lymphoma with a very low ADC value (0.65   10 ^{3} mm^2/s). (b) A lymph node in squamous cell carcinoma with a slightly higher ADC value (1.0   10 ^{3} mm^2/s).

necrosis and perfusion between cancers that can be detected by DWI and used to characterize lymphadenopathy. In the case of SCC, diffusion is less restricted than in lymphoma, and hence the ADC values of SCC nodes are higher [29,30] (Fig. 7.6). Recent work suggests that there are differences also in the ADC value between benign and malignant cervical nodes, as well as between nodes containing different histological tumor types [30,31].

Dynamic contrast-enhanced imaging
Low-molecular-weight paramagnetic contrast agents such as gadolinium can be used to assess the microvasculature and the extravascular extracellular space of nodal cancers. In the head and neck region, rapid serial imaging is performed using T_1-weighted gradient echo images as the intravenous contrast passes through the node. The results are analyzed using time–signal intensity plots or pharmacokinetic models (Fig. 7.7.). Early work suggests that there may be a difference in the contrast enhancement of metastatic and normal nodes, the latter showing a shorter time to peak, higher peak enhancement and faster wash-out phase [32]. The enhancement pattern also shows promise in predicting local control in head and neck cancers [33,34].

Proton magnetic resonance spectroscopy
Proton spectroscopy can demonstrate choline at 3.2 ppm in nodal metastases from HNSCC [35] (Fig. 7.8). At present the role of MRS in identifying metastatic nodes is

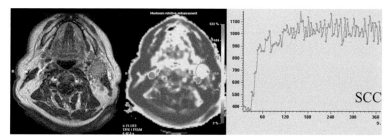

Fig. 7.7. Dynamic contrast-enhanced MRI of metastatic node in squamous cell carcinoma, with the corresponding time–signal intensity curve. Color version in plate section.

limited by technical difficulties, including the relatively large volume of tissue required for successful analysis (1 cm^3) and long acquisition time.

Ultrasmall super paramagnetic iron oxide particles

Iron particles injected intravenously are taken up by macrophages in normally functioning nodes. This results in a decrease in the T_2-weighted signal intensity of normal nodes while metastatic nodes retain the signal intensity. This technique produces negative predictive values of $\leqslant 90\%$ and positive predictive values of $\leqslant 51\%$, but it is hampered by movement and susceptibility artefacts and it requires two MRI examinations, one before and one 24–36 h after administration of the particles [36].

Distant disease spread

Incidence and sites of spread

Improvements in locoregional control of SCC have lead to distant disease spread becoming a common cause of mortality. Distant metastases from SCC are found in approximately 7–17% of patients with advanced stage disease at diagnosis [37,38], but up to 25% of patients eventually develop metastases. This figure rises to more than 50% when results from autopsy series are taken into account. Around 80% of clinically detected metastases arise in the first 2 years after diagnosis, with the majority occurring in the first 12–15 months. Once distant metastases occur, survival is usually less than 1 year [39]. The majority of distant metastases are found in the chest, involving the lungs (80%) or mediastinal nodes (34%). The next most common sites are bone and liver, which tend to occur in the presence of chest metastases. Following treatment, distant metastases may be found at unusual sites such as the skin, bone marrow and nodes in the axillary, inguinal and intercostal regions.

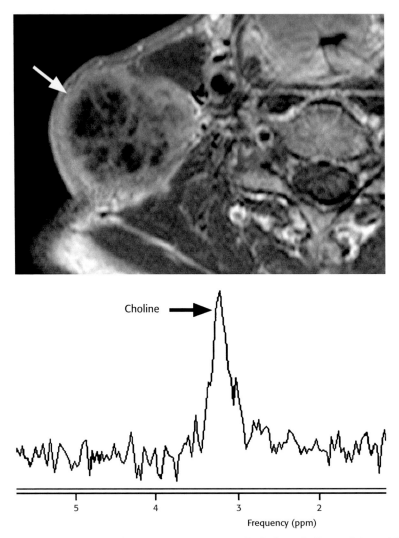

Fig. 7.8. Proton magnetic resonance spectroscopy displaying a choline peak (arrow) in a metastatic node (arrow) from squamous cell carcinoma.

Imaging distant metastases

The chest radiograph is routinely used in all patients to screen the chest for distant metastases and synchronous primary lung cancers, but it has a low sensitivity compared with a CT of the thorax (sensitivity for the chest radiograph ranges from 21 to 50%) [40,41] (Fig. 7.9). Therefore a CT of the thorax is performed in those patients considered to be at "high risk" of distant metastases. One of the most

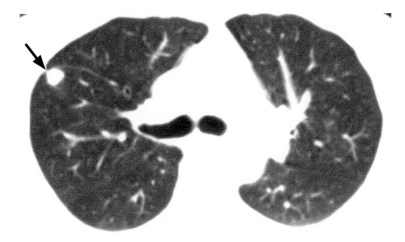

Fig. 7.9. A CT image of the thorax (lung window) of a patient with a hypopharyngeal squamous cell carcinoma who has a second primary cancer in the lung (arrow), which was missed on the chest radiograph.

important factors for high risk of distant metastases is advanced nodal disease. This high-risk group includes patients with large nodes (>6 cm), multiple nodes (>3), nodes with ENS, and nodes involving the lower neck/supraclavicular fossa [38,40,42,43] (Fig. 7.10). Other considerations are (a) the primary tumor, including advanced/large cancers, poorly differentiated cancers and those that arise from primary sites in the hypopharynx, base of tongue and supraglottic larynx; (b) second primary tumors; and (c) locoregional recurrence. Apart from "high risk cancers," CT of the thorax may be performed for clinical trials and in those patients in whom extensive and potentially mutilating surgery is planned in the neck.

Imaging at sites outside the chest is performed according to clinical and biochemical findings, although blood biochemistry for liver and bone disease is unreliable. Liver metastases are found in as many as 31% of patients at autopsy [44], but imaging detection is uncommon and does not appear to be justified, especially where there is no evidence of chest metastases. However, when a CT of the thorax is performed for chest metastases, the scan is usually extended to include the entire liver in one examination [38,40,45]. Bone metastases are found with a similar frequency to liver metastases at autopsy [44], but once again clinical detection is low, at only 4% [38]. Bone metastases most commonly involve the thoracic and lumbar spine, followed by ribs, and therefore some will be detectable on a CT of the thorax (Fig. 7.11). The bone scan is a very sensitive technique for detecting bone metastases but it has a high incidence of false-positive results and the

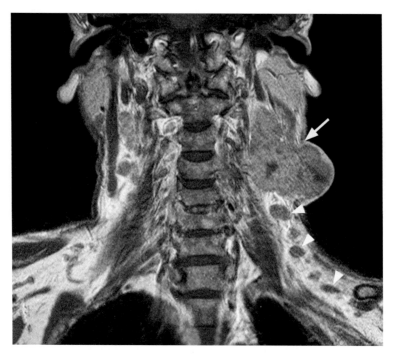

Fig. 7.10. Coronal contrast-enhanced T$_1$-weighted MRI showing a bulky metastatic node (arrow) and multiple nodes extending down to the lower neck (arrowheads) in a patient with a hypopharyngeal squamous cell carcinoma who later developed mediastinal nodal and pulmonary metastases.

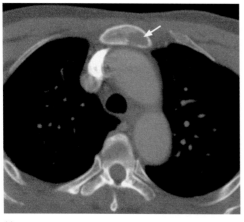

(a)

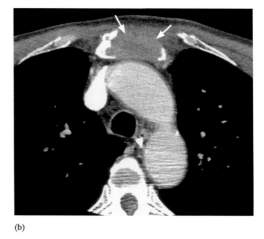

(b)

Fig 7.11. Thoracic CT in a patient with a hypopharyngeal squamous cell carcinoma (SCC). (a) There is a bone metastasis in the sternum (arrow) at the time of diagnosis (bone window). (b) This has increased in size 6 months after treatment of SCC (mediastinal window).

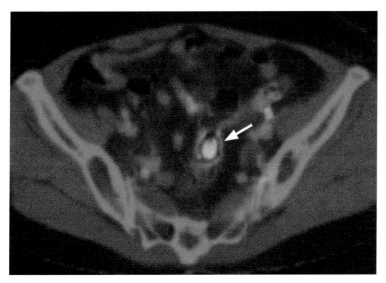

Fig. 7.12. Early adenocarcinoma of the sigmoid colon (arrow) detected by ¹⁸F-Fluorodeoxyglucose PET, which was performed to screen for distant metastases from a primary nasopharyngeal carcinoma. Color version in plate section.

additional costs of confirming the nature of the abnormalities on the bone scan do not appear to justify its routine use [38].

Unfortunately, 11% of patients with a negative CT of the thorax go on to develop distant metastases in the chest or elsewhere within 12 months, leading Brouwer *et al.* to propose that a whole-body imaging technique is required [46]. At present, FDG PET has not been shown to be of value for detecting distant metastases from HNSCC compared with other imaging techniques [47]. In the chest, it has problems detecting lung tumors < 1 cm in size [48], although it does appear to have some advantages in detecting mediastinal nodes [49,50]. Inflammation also leads to false-positive results with FDG PET, not only in the chest but also at other sites in the body [47,51]. Interestingly, one of the main advantages of FDG PET appears to be the detection of unsuspected second primary cancers. Patients with HNSCC often have a history of smoking and high alcohol intake, which exposes them to an increased risk of other cancers. Synchronous tumors (within 6 months) are believed to occur in about 4% of patients [52], but the incidence increases for metachronous cancers (after 6 months). Use of FDG PET has shown an even higher incidence of synchronous tumors, reported in 6–18% of patients [47,53,54]. These second primary cancers involve not only the chest and upper areodigestive tract but also sites such as the lower gastrointestinal tract and the liver (Fig. 7.12). In patients with early-stage HNSCC, these second primary cancers are a leading cause of death. This finding raises the interesting dilemma of whether FDG PET should be considered in both early- and advanced-stage HNSCC.

Conclusions

The modality of choice for staging HNSCC nodes is dictated by the primary tumor and, therefore, it usually lies between MRI or CT. Overall, there is little difference in these two techniques for evaluating nodes, except with respect to retropharyngeal nodes, where MRI has the advantage. Ultrasound has some advantages over MRI/ CT in demonstrating the nodal hilum and vascular pattern, as well as for image-guided biopsy. Ultrasound is of most value when used in patients in whom MRI/CT staging has shown indeterminate nodes or an N0 neck. It is also the primary imaging technique for follow-up of patients with an N0 neck who undergo a "wait and see" approach rather than elective surgery. The role of functional imaging is still evolving, with FDG PET being the most widely used functional technique as nodal metastases from SCC are FDG avid. The technique appears to perform as well as or slightly better than the morphological techniques, but it too has problems with false-positive and false-negative results.

Advanced nodal disease is one of the most important indicators for distant metastases. The chest is the most common site for these metastases but because the sensitivity of the chest radiograph is low, a CT of the thorax is indicated in patients considered to be at high risk. Unfortunately, some patients with a normal CT of the thorax go on to develop distant metastases in the chest or elsewhere within 12 months. The best method for detecting these early distant metastases has not been established and as yet the role of FDG PET is unknown. However, early results show that FDG PET may be of value in detecting unsuspected synchronous tumors.

REFERENCES

1. H. Rouvière. *Lymphatic System of the Head and Neck*. (Ann Arbor, MI: Edwards Brothers, 1938).
2. J. P. Shah, E. Strong, R. H. Spiro, *et al.* Surgical grand rounds: neck dissection – current status and future possibilities. *Clin Bull* **11** (1981), 25–33.
3. K. T. Robbins, G. Clayman, P. A. Levine, For the American Head and Neck Society, American Academy of Otolaryngology-Head and Neck Surgery. Neck dissection classification update:

revisions proposed by the American Head and Neck Society and the American Academy of Otolaryngology-Head and Neck Surgery. *Arch Otolaryngol Head Neck Surg* **128** (2002), 751–758.

4. P. M. Som, H. D. Curtin, A. A. Mancuso. Imaging-based classification for evaluation of neck metastatic adenopathy. *Am J Roentgenol* **174** (2000), 837–844.

5. P. Levendag, M. Braaksma, E. Coche, *et al*. Rotterdam and Brussels CT-based neck nodal delineation compared with the surgical levels as defined by the American Academy of Otolaryngology-Head and Neck Surgery. *Int J Radiat Oncol Biol Phys* **58** (2004), 113–123.

6. F. L. Greene, D. L. Page, I. D. Fleming, *et al*. *AJCC Cancer Staging Manual* 6th edn. (New York: Springer-Verlag, 2002).

7. H. D. Curtin, H. Ishwaran, A. A. Mancuso, *et al*. Comparison of CT and MR imaging in staging of neck metastases. *Radiology* **207** (1998), 123–130.

8. M. W. M. van der Brekel, H. V. Stel, J. A. Castelijns, *et al*. Cervical lymph node metastasis: assessment of radiologic criteria. *Radiology* **177** (1990), 379–384.

9. M. W. M. van den Brekel, J. A. Castelijns, G. B. Snow. The size of lymph nodes in the neck on sonograms as a radiologic criterion for metastasis: how reliable is it? *Am J Neuroradiol* **19** (1998), 695–700.

10. H. J. Steinkamp, M. Cornehl, N. Hosten, *et al*. Cervical lymphadenopathy: ratio of long to short-axis diameter as a predictor of malignancy. *Br J Radiol* **68** (1995), 266–270.

11. A. D. King, G. M. K. Tse, A. T. Ahuja, *et al*. Comparison of the diagnostic accuracy of CT, MR imaging and US for the detection of necrosis in metastatic neck nodes. *Radiology* **230** (2004), 720–726.

12. A. D. King, G. M. K. Tse, E. H. Y. Yuen, *et al*. Comparison of CT and MR imaging for the detection of extranodal neoplastic spread in metastatic neck nodes. *Eur J Radiol* **52** (2004), 264–270.

13. M. Ying, A. T. Ahuja, F. Brook, C. Metreweli. Vascularity and grey-scale sonographic features of normal cervical lymph nodes: variations with nodal size. *Clin Radiol* **56** (2001), 416–419.

14. A. T. Ahuja, M. Ying, A. D. King, E. H. Y. Yuen. Lymph node hilus: gray scale and power Doppler sonography of cervical nodes. *J Ultrasound Med* **20** (2001), 987–992.

15. A. T. Ahuja, M. Ying, S. S. Ho, C. Metreweli. Distribution of intranodal vessels in differentiating benign from metastatic nodes. *Clin Radiol* **56** (2001), 197–201.

16. M. W. M. van den Brekel, J. A. Castelijns, H. V. Stel, *et al*. Occult metastatic neck disease: detection with US and US-guided fine-needle aspiration cytology. *Radiology* **180** (1991), 457–461.

17. J. A. Castelijns, M. W. M. van den Brekel. Imaging of lymphadenopathy in the neck. *Eur Radiol* **12** (2002), 727–738.

18. M. W. M. van den Brekel, J. A. Castelijns, H. V. Stel, *et al*. Modern imaging techniques and ultrasound-guided aspiration cytology for the assessment of neck node metastases: a prospective comparative study. *Eur Arch Otorhinolaryngol* **250** (1993), 11–17.

19. T. S. Atula, M. J. Varpula, T. J. I. Kurki, P. J. Klemi, R. Grénman. Assessment of cervical lymph node status in head and neck cancer patients: palpation, computed tomography and low field magnetic resonance imaging compared with ultrasound-guided fine-needle aspiration cytology. *Eur J Radiol* **25** (1997), 152–161.

20. T. Stuckensen, A. F. Kovács, S. Adams, R. P. Baum. Staging of the neck in patients with oral cavity squamous cell carcinomas: a prospective comparison of PET, ultrasound, CT and MRI. *J Craniomaxillofac Surg* **28** (2000), 319–324.

21. R. B. J. de Bondt, P. J. Nelemans, P. A. M. Hofman, *et al*. Detection of lymph node metastases in head and neck cancer: a meta-analysis comparing US, USgFNAC, CT and MR imaging. *Eur J Radiol* **64** (2007), 266–272.

22. M. H. Weiss, L. B. Harrison, R. S. Isaacs. Use of decision analysis in planning a management strategy for the stage N0 neck. *Arch Otolaryngol Head Neck Surg* **120** (1994), 699–702.

23. C. G. Gourin. Is selective neck dissection adequate treatment for node-positive disease? *Arch Otolaryngol Head Neck Surg* **130** (2004), 1431–1434.

24. M. W. M. van den Brekel, J. A. Castelijns, L. C. Reitsma, *et al*. Outcome of observing the N0 neck using ultrasonographic-guided cytology for follow-up. *Arch Otolaryngol Head Neck Surg* **125** (1999), 153–156.

25. D. J. Adelstein, J. P. Saxton, L. A. Rybicki, *et al*. Multiagent concurrent chemoradiotherapy for locoregionally advanced squamous cell head and neck cancer: mature results from a single institution. *J Clin Oncol* **24** (2006), 1064–1071.

26. H. Schoder, H. W. Yeung. Positron emission imaging of head and neck cancer, including thyroid carcinoma. *Semin Nucl Med* **34** (2004), 180–197.

27. J. W. Braams, J. Pruim, N. J. M. Freling, *et al*. Detection of lymph node metastases of squamous-cell cancer of the head and neck with FDG-PET and MRI. *J Nucl Med* **36** (1995), 211–216.

28. Y. Kitagawa, K. Sano, S. Nishizawa, *et al*. FDG-PET for prediction of tumor aggressiveness and response to intra-arterial chemotherapy and radiotherapy in head and neck cancer. *Eur J Nucl Med Mol Imaging* **30** (2003), 63–71.

29. M. Maeda, H. Kato, H. Sakuma, S. E. Maier, K. Takeda. Usefulness of the apparent diffusion coefficient in line scan diffusion-weighted imaging for distinguishing between squamous cell carcinomas and malignant lymphomas of the head and neck. *Am J Neuroradiol* **26** (2005), 1186–1192.

30. A. A. Abdel Razek, N. Y. Soliman, S. Elkhamary, M. K. Alsharaway, A. Tawfik. Role of diffusion-weighted MR imaging in cervical lymphadenopathy. *Eur Radiol* **16** (2006), 1468–1477.

31. A. D. King, A. T. Ahuja, D. K. Yeung, *et al*. Malignant cervical lymphadenopathy: diagnostic accuracy of diffusion-weighted MRI imaging. *Radiology* **245** (2007), 806–813.

32. N. J. Fischbein, S. M. Noworolski, R. G. Henry, *et al*. Assessment of metastatic cervical adenopathy using dynamic contrast-enhanced MR imaging. *Am J Neuroradiol* **24** (2003), 301–311.

33. N. Tomura, K. Omachi, I. Sakuma, *et al*. Dynamic contrast-enhanced magnetic resonance imaging in radiotherapeutic efficacy in the head and neck tumors. *Am J Otolaryngol* **26** (2005), 163–167.

34. P. J. Hoskin, M. I. Saunders, K. Goodchild, *et al*. Dynamic contrast enhanced magnetic resonance scanning as a predictor of response to accelerated radiotherapy for advanced head and neck cancer. *Br J Radiol* **72** (1999), 1093–1098.

35. S. K. Mukherji, S. Schiro, M. Castillo, *et al.* Proton MR spectroscopy of squamous cell carcinoma of the extracranial head and neck. *Am J Neuroradiol* **18** (1997), 1057–1072.

36. R. Sigal, T. Vogl, J. Casselman, *et al.* Lymph node metastases from head and neck squamous cell carcinoma: MR imaging with ultrasmall superparamagnetic iron oxide particles (Sinerem MR) – results of a phase III multicenter clinical trial. *Eur Radiol* **12** (2002), 1104–1113.

37. M. L. Dennington, D. R. Carter, A. D. Meyers. Distant metastases in head and neck epidermoid carcinoma. *Laryngoscope* **90** (1980), 196–201.

38. R. de Bree, E. E. Deurloo, G. B. Snow, C. R. Leemans. Screening for distant metastases in patients with head and neck cancer. *Laryngoscope* **110** (2000), 397–401.

39. K. H. Calhourn, P. Fulmer, R. Weiss, J. A. Hokanson. Distant metastases from head and neck squamous cell carcinomas. *Laryngoscope* **104** (1994), 1199–1205.

40. D. J. Houghton, M. L. Hughes, C. Garvey, *et al.* Role of chest CT scanning in the management of patients presenting with head and neck cancer. *Head Neck* **20** (1998), 614–618.

41. R. J. Troell, D. J. Terris. Detection of metastases from head and neck cancers. *Laryngoscope* **105** (1995), 247–250.

42. C. R. Leemans, R. Tiwari, J. J. P. Nauta, I. van der Waal, G. B. Snow. Regional lymph node involvement and its significance in the development of distant metastases in head and neck carcinoma. *Cancer* **71** (1993), 452–456.

43. A. Alvi, J. T. Johnson. Development of distant metastasis after treatment of advanced-stage head and neck cancer. *Head Neck* **19** (1997), 500–505.

44. C. Kotwall, K. Sako, M. S. Razack, U. Rao, V. Bakamjian, D. P. Shedd. Metastatic patterns in squamous cell cancer of the head and neck. *Am J Surg* **154** (1987), 439–442.

45. B. Reiner, E. Siegel, R. Sawyer, *et al.* The impact of routine CT of the chest on the diagnosis and management of newly diagnosed squamous cell carcinoma of the head and neck. *Am J Roentgenol* **169** (1997), 667–671.

46. J. Brouwer, R. de Bree, O. S. Hoekstra, *et al.* Screening for distant metastases in patients with head and neck cancer: is chest computed tomography sufficient? *Laryngoscope* **115** (2005), 1813–1817.

47. J. Brouwer, A. Senft, R. de Bree, *et al.* Screening for distant metastases in patients with head and neck cancer: is there a role for (18)FDG-PET? *Oral Oncol* **42** (2006), 275–280.

48. J. F. Vansteenkiste. Imaging in lung cancer: positron emission tomography scan. *Eur Respir J* **19** (2002), 49–60.

49. D. L. Schwartz, J. Rajendran, B. Yueh, *et al.* Staging of head and neck squamous cell cancer with extended-field FDG-PET. *Arch Otolaryngol Head Neck Surg* **129** (2003), 1173–1178.

50. T. N. Teknos, E. L. Rosenthal, D. Lee, R. Taylor, C. S. Marn. Positron emission tomography in the evaluation of stage III and IV head and neck cancer. *Head Neck* **23** (2001), 1056–1060.

51. J. W. Keyes, M. Y. Chen, N. E. Watson, *et al.* FDG PET evaluation of head and neck cancer: value of imaging the thorax. *Head Neck* **22** (2000), 105–110.

52. B. H. Haughey, G. A. Gates, C. L. Arfken, J. H. Harvey. Meta-analysis of second malignant tumors in head and neck cancer: the case for an endoscopic screening protocol. *Ann Otol Rhinol Laryngol* **101** (1992), 105–112.

53. G. W. Goerres, D. T. Schmid, K. W. Gratz, G. K. von Schulthess, G. K. Eyrich. Impact of whole body positron emission tomography on initial staging and therapy in patients with squamous cell carcinoma of the oral cavity. *Oral Oncol* **39** (2003), 547–551.

54. M. P. M. Stokkel, K. G. M. Moons, F. W. ten Broek, P. P. van Rijk, G. J. Hordijk. ^{18}F-fluorodeoxyglucose dual-head positron emission tomography as a procedure for detecting simultaneous primary tumors in cases of head and neck. *Cancer* **86** (2000), 2370–2377.

8

Post-treatment imaging

Robert Hermans

Introduction

Post-treatment imaging is carried out when a recurrent tumor is suspected, to confirm the presence of such a lesion and to determine its extent. The extent of a recurrent cancer is important information for determining the possibility of salvage therapy.

Imaging may also be used to monitor tumor response and to try to detect recurrent or persistent disease before it becomes clinically evident, possibly with a better chance for successful salvage. However, early tumor recurrence may be difficult to distinguish from tissue changes induced by therapy. Therefore, the expected changes on imaging studies after treatment of a head and neck cancer should be clearly understood when analyzing images.

Treatment complications are less frequent than tumor recurrences, but these conditions may sometimes be clinically difficult to distinguish. Although definitive distinction between treatment-induced necrosis and recurrent tumor may also be difficult radiologically, imaging findings may be helpful in guiding treatment and assessing response to specific treatment.

Expected tissue changes after radiotherapy

The changes visible on post-treatment computed tomography (CT) and magnetic resonance imaging (MRI) depend on the radiation dose and rate, the irradiated tissue volume and the time elapsed since the end of radiation therapy [1]. Changes which may be seen include (Fig. 8.1):

thickening of the skin and platysma muscle

reticulation of the subcutaneous fat and the deep tissue fat layers

edema in the retropharyngeal space

increased enhancement of the major salivary glands, followed by size reduction of these glands: postirradiation sialadenitis

Squamous Cell Cancer of the Neck, ed. Robert Hermans. Published by Cambridge University Press.
© R. Hermans 2009.

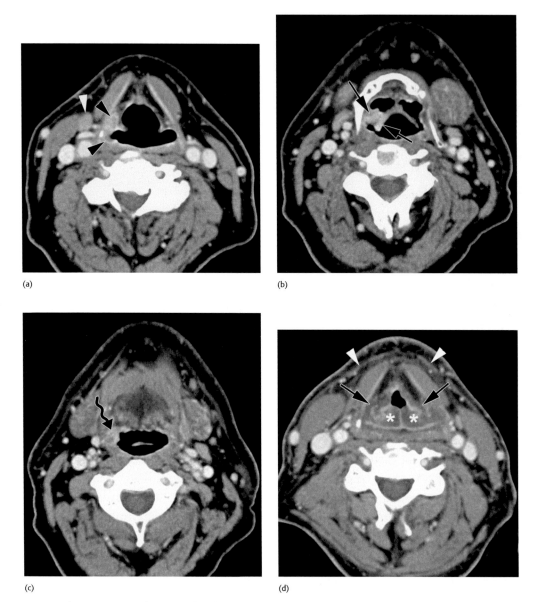

(a)

(b)

(c)

(d)

Fig. 8.1. Computed tomography of a patient suffering squamous cell cancer in the right pyriform sinus before (a–c) and 4 months after the end of chemoradiotherapy (d–f). (a–c) The tumor is growing in the paraglottic space (black arrowheads) and extends along the pharyngo-epiglottic fold (arrows) in the posterolateral border of the tongue base (curved arrow). Radiological staging is T4a, N1. (d–f) Radiation-induced soft tissue swelling is noted, particularly at the level of the aryepiglottic folds (asterisks). Increased attenuation of the fat is seen (black arrows). At the level of the tumor bed, the larynx, hypopharynx and tongue base appear symmetrical, indicating a favorable response to treatment. Extralaryngeal/extrapharyngeal tissue changes include thickening of the platysma muscles (arrowheads), and volume loss and increased enhancement of the submandibular salivary glands (white arrows). The lymph node, visible before treatment, is not seen any more. This patient is without evidence of locoregional disease 2 years after treatment.

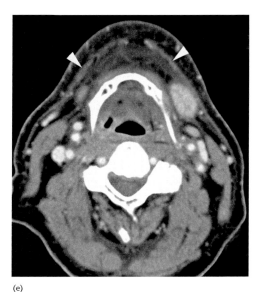 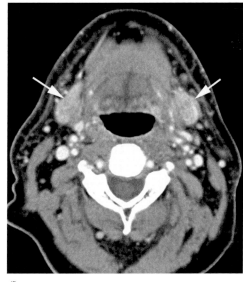

(e)   (f)

Fig 8.1. (cont.)

atrophy of lymphatic tissue, in both the lymph nodes and Waldeyer's ring
thickening and increased enhancement of the pharyngeal walls
thickening of the laryngeal structures.

These tissue changes are most pronounced during the first few months after the end
of radiation therapy, and diminish or even resolve with time. These expected tissue
changes after radiation therapy appear symmetrical, unless the neck was irradiated
using asymmetric radiation portals.

Expected tissue changes after surgery

The limits of surgical therapy are determined by the balance between radical
resection of the tumor and leaving the patient in a functionally and esthetically
acceptable situation. More extensive resections are possible by the introduction of
various reconstructive materials, such as pedicled or free soft tissue flaps, grafts and
prostheses.

The most commonly used pedicled flap is the pectoralis major flap. It is commonly used to reconstruct the pharyngeal defect after laryngectomy with partial
pharyngectomy; it is also very useful for closing defects in the irradiated neck, as it
introduces tissue with a fresh blood supply.

On imaging studies, the pectoralis major flap appears initially as a bulky soft tissue structure, showing the characteristics of muscle; gradually, denervation atrophy appears, causing volume loss and fatty replacement of the muscle.

When a flap is vascularized by local vessels, anastomosed to the flap by micro-vascular techniques, it is called a free flap. Different kinds of free flap are in use, for example cutaneous flaps to reconstruct defects in the oral cavity, osseous flaps (e.g., fibula) to reconstruct mandibular defects, and free jejunal interposition to recon-struct the defect created by a total laryngopharyngectomy.

Neck dissection is a surgical procedure to remove neck nodal metastases. Several procedures are distinguished. In radical neck dissection, unilateral en bloc removal of the neck lymph nodes levels I to V [2], including the sternocleidomastoid muscle, internal jugular vein, submandibular gland and spinal accessory nerve, is per-formed. If the spinal accessory nerve is preserved, the procedure is called a modified radical neck dissection.

If the spinal accessory nerve and one or more of the above mentioned structures, removed in a radical neck dissection, is preserved, the procedure is called a func-tional or conservative neck dissection. This type of dissection is performed when there are no, or only small, clinically or radiographically positive lymph nodes present in the neck.

In a selective neck dissection, a more limited number of lymph node levels are removed. A commonly performed selective neck dissection is a supraomohyoid neck dissection: this includes removal of levels I, II and III.

Surveillance imaging of the primary tumor site

In most patients, CT is an adequate imaging modality for pre- and post-treatment imaging; MRI is preferred in patients with nasopharyngeal, sinonasal and skull base tumors.

After radiation therapy, tumor recurrence appears on CT or MRI as a soft tissue mass at the primary site. After surgery, tumor recurrence typically appears as a soft tissue mass along the resection margins. Bone or cartilage erosion may be seen in large recurrent tumors. Also perivascular or perineural spread may be seen on imaging studies.

Early tumor recurrence may be difficult to distinguish from tissue changes induced by therapy. Therefore, it is recommended to obtain a follow-up CT or MRI study after surgical, radiation or combined treatment for a head and neck neoplasm with a high-risk profile [3,4]. Probably the best time to obtain such a

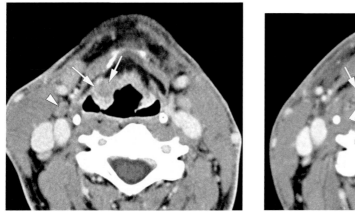
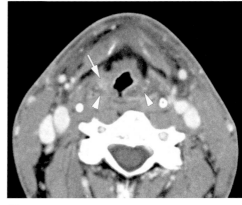

(a)

(b)

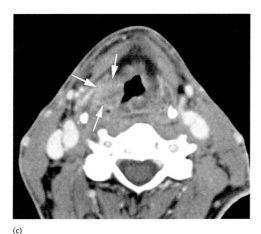

(c)

Fig. 8.2. Axial contrast-enhanced CT images in a patient with supraglottic cancer. (a) Pretreatment image. A right-sided, enhancing infiltrating soft tissue mass can be seen in the supraglottis (arrow). There is a small metastatic lymph node (arrowhead). (b) Baseline follow-up, 4 months after radiotherapy. Clinically, there is no evidence of disease. The thickening and increased attenuation of the aryepiglottic folds is an expected finding (arrowheads). However, the asymmetrical and slightly enhancing tissue infiltration in the tumor bed (arrow) is doubtful. Follow-up CT study was recommended. (c) At 8 months after the end of radiotherapy, the patient reported some pain and swallowing difficulties, but clinical examination did not reveal any abnormalities. On CT, the soft-tissue infiltration in the supraglottis (arrows) is progressive compared with the baseline study, highly suspect for tumor recurrence. Direct laryngoscopy was performed, showing an intact mucosa; biopsy at the suspect area was negative. Repeat direct laryngoscopy and deep (submucosal) tissue biopsies confirmed the presence of cancer. Subsequently, a total laryngectomy was performed.

baseline study is about 3–6 months after the end of treatment. Such a baseline study documents treatment-caused changes in the head and neck tissues. By comparing subsequent studies with the baseline study, tumor recurrences or treatment complications can be detected with more confidence, and often at an earlier stage than by clinical follow-up alone (Fig. 8.2).

The baseline study itself carries important predictive information regarding the eventual local outcome: CT achieves a sensitivity of 83% and a specificity of 95% in the early differentiation of treatment responders from non-responders in irradiated laryngeal and hypopharyngeal cancer [3]. In advanced head and neck cancer, treated by chemoradiation, MRI performed 6 to 8 weeks after the end of treatment was able to predict residual/recurrent disease at the primary site with a sensitivity of 48% and a specificity of 85% [5]. In this same study, it was shown that a clinical examination of the head and neck under general anesthesia, at the same time points, had limited value, as most local recurrences remained undetected. These authors recommended the performance of such an endoscopic examination only in patients with suspect findings on early follow-up MRI [5].

Some authors recommend positon emission tomography (PET) with ^{18}F-fluorodeoxyglucose (FDG) as the initial baseline study [6]. If performed 3–4 months after treatment, the negative predictive value of PET is consistently high. However, false-negative results occasionally occur, owing to the low spatial resolution of PET. The positive predictive value of post-treatment PET is clearly lower, as possible false-positive results occur because of therapy-induced inflammatory changes. A positive post-treatment PET study should be correlated with the clinical findings and results from other imaging modalities, and histological examination is required (Fig. 8.3). In case of a negative biopsy, close follow-up is recommended [7].

Relatively few studies are available that prospectively compare dedicated CT or MRI of the head and neck with PET in the post-treatment situation. Somewhat better results have been reported with PET than with CT and/or MRI [8,9].

It has been suggested that combined PET/CT is superior to CT after chemoradiotherapy [10], but in this study the CT portion of the PET/CT study was compared with the combined information from both modalities. The diagnostic yield of the CT portion of such a combined study is inherently limited by technical factors, such as patient positioning, contrast-injection protocol and slice thickness. The CT portion of such a combined study is helpful to correct the shortcomings of PET [11], but cannot be expected to provide similar diagnostic information as a dedicated CT study of the head and neck.

A technique that has recently been introduced in the evaluation of head and neck cancer is diffusion-weighted MRI. This provides information about microscopic structures such as cell density, cell integrity and vascularity, and is applicable in the head and neck region [12–14]. This technique is very sensitive to structural changes in pathological tissue, even during their very early stages of development. As it is a completely non-invasive technique, not requiring an external contrast agent,

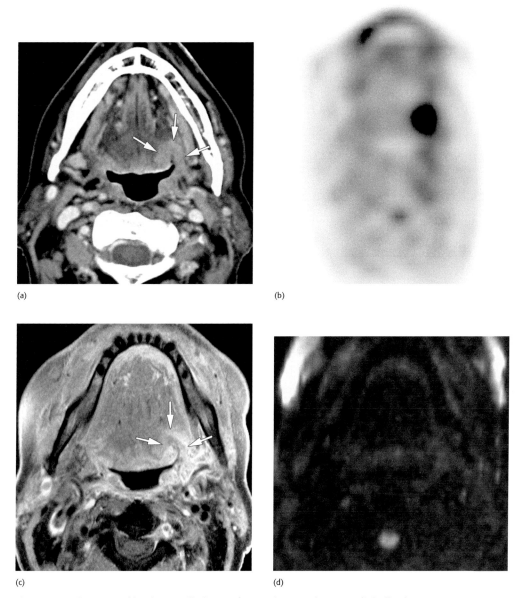

(a)

(b)

(c)

(d)

Fig. 8.3. A patient treated by chemoradiotherapy for oropharyngeal cancer. Clinically, there was persistent and painful soft tissue thickening and ulceration at the site of the primary tumor. (a) Axial contrast-enhanced CT, obtained 4 months after the end of treatment, shows an ulcerated soft tissue mass (arrows) in the base of the tongue, corresponding to the pretreatment position of the primary tumor, which raises suspicion of persisting tumor. (b) An axial ^{18}F-fluorodeoxyglucose PET image, obtained 3 weeks later, shows a hot spot, anatomically corresponding to the lesion on the tongue base: this is compatible with persisting tumor. (c) An axial gadolinium-enhanced T_1-weighted spin-echo image, obtained 1 week after (b), confirms a lesion (arrows) in the tongue base, essentially showing similar abnormalities to the CT image. (d) A diffusion-weighted image (b1000) shows uniform low signal intensity in the tongue base. (e) The corresponding (ADC) map apparent diffusion coefficient reveals high values in the tissue surrounding the ulceration (arrows), indicating absence of diffusion restriction (ADC was 167 10^{-5} mm^2/s). The findings in (d) and (e) are not compatible with residual tumor but indicate inflammation and/or necrosis. Surgical resection was performed. Histological examination showed a necrotic ulcer with surrounding inflammation; no residual tumor was found.

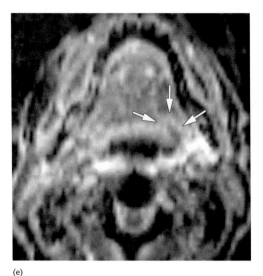

Fig. 8.3. (cont.)

(e)

diffusion-weighted MRI potentially has important advantages for evaluating the head and neck after treatment. Initial results suggest that this technique may be more specific than FDG PET (Fig. 8.3) [14].

Imaging of nodal disease after (chemo)radiotherapy

Patients with advanced head and neck cancer, treated by (chemo)radiotherapy, may show persisting nodal disease at the end of treatment. In such patients, the role of surgery (i.e., a planned neck dissection) is not well defined [15]. Such a planned neck dissection may reduce the regional failure rate and improve survival. However, many of these neck resection specimens do not contain tumor, meaning that the patient was exposed to the inherent risks of surgery without benefit.

Using CT of the neck early after the end of (chemo)radiotherapy has been shown to be a reliable method to predict the absence of residual nodal disease. Absence of lymph nodes > 1.5 cm and lack of any focal nodal abnormality had a negative predictive value of 94%, while that of the clinical evaluation was 77% [16]. However, both the clinical examination and CT have a poor positive predictive value of approximately 40%; this means that many patients with positive findings will eventually not show regional tumor recurrence (Fig. 8.4).

As for the primary tumor site, FDG PET is recommended by some authors for detecting residual nodal disease. However, FDG PET obtained early after the end of therapy appears to be unreliable. In a prospective study on 12 patients treated by

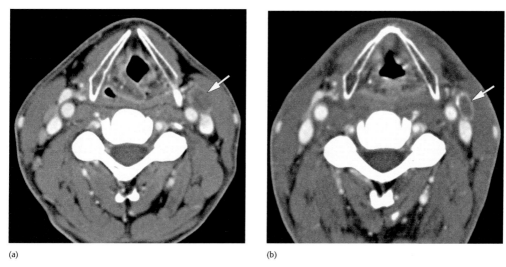

(a)   (b)

Fig. 8.4. A patient suffering oropharyngeal cancer, staged as T4a N2c. (a) Axial contrast-enhanced CT image obtained before therapy shows centrally necrotic adenopathy in level III on the left side (arrow). (b) A CT image was obtained 2 months after end of chemoradiotherapy. The primary tumor (not shown) responded well to treatment. The adenopathy was only slightly diminished in size (diameter approximately 1.4 cm, arrow). A wait-and-see policy was adopted, and no neck dissection was performed. The adenopathy gradually decreased in size on follow-up CT studies. There was no evidence of disease 4 years after the end of treatment.

radiotherapy alone, a negative predictive value of 14% was obtained when PET was done 1 month after treatment [17]. This high level of false-negative findings may be related to temporary changes in tumor glucose metabolism induced by therapy [18]. More reliable results are obtained when FDG PET is performed 3–4 months after the end of treatment, resulting in a negative predictive value of 97–100% [19,20].

Also for this indication, preliminary results indicate that diffusion-weighted-MRI may be a valuable method to select patients who may benefit from an added neck dissection [14].

Impact of post-treatment imaging on patient survival

Currently, few data regarding the impact of post-treatment surveillance on patient survival are available. Some authors argue that routine follow-up is indispensable, as patients with asymptomatic locoregional recurrences, discovered during surveillance, have a significantly better postrecurrence survival than those patients where recurrent disease was found by symptoms [21]. Other authors point out that the apparently longer survival of patients with recurrent tumor diagnosed by testing may be a result of lead time bias (i.e., early diagnosis falsely appears to prolong survival) [4]. This statement probably is true for patients treated by combined-modality therapy for advanced head and neck cancer, who are known to do extremely poorly after relapse and rarely have an effective treatment option available [22]. However, in patients treated by a single modality, where a reasonable chance of salvage exists after loco-regional recurrence (e.g. 35–60% surgical salvage rate for irradiated laryngeal cancer), imaging surveillance may be worthwhile to add to the clinical follow-up in order to further improve the salvage rate. More studies are required to elucidate this question.

Treatment complications

Complications after surgery

Most surgical complications occur early after treatment and are dealt with on a clinical basis. Imaging may be required in the detection and visualization of a fistula originating from the oral cavity or pharynx. Many of these fistulas will close sponta-neously, but some may need reintervention. Imaging may also be of use in the confirmation of flap failure through necrosis.

Complications after radiotherapy

Acute effects of radiotherapy (skin and mucosal reactions) occur during or imme-diately after treatment and usually settle spontaneously.

Tissue necrosis is a rare complication of radiotherapy in the head and neck region, usually appearing months to years after the end of radiation treatment. Several risk factors have been identified, including high radiation doses and large radiation fields. Soft tissue, cartilage and bone necrosis may be encountered and several tissue types may be involved at the same time.

Mandibular osteoradionecrosis
Mandibular osteoradionecrosis is a rare but feared complication as it may interfere with basic physiological functions, such as swallowing and breathing. Trauma (e.g., dental surgery) is often associated with the appearance of osteoradionecrosis as it creates a demand for tissue repair beyond the capabilities of the irradiated tissue [23].

The CT findings include bony abnormalities (cortical interruptions and loss of spongiosa trabeculation), sequestration, pathological fractures, soft tissue thicken-ing (sometimes containing gas) and fistula formation (Fig. 8.5). Radiologically, differentiation from tumor recurrence may be difficult. In the mandible, some

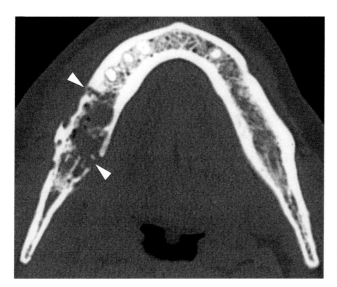

Fig. 8.5. Axial CT image (bone window) of a patient treated 10 years earlier by external irradiation for a right-sided parotid malignancy and who now presented with oral pain and mucosal dehiscence. Extensive resorption of spongiosa in the right mandibular body (compare with opposite side), and destruction of both lingual and buccal cortex can be seen, complicated by a pathological fracture (arrowheads). Intra-osseous air bubbles can be seen. Histopathological study showed necrotic bone with signs of osteomyelitis.

findings, such as the association with cortical defects away from the position of the original tumor (at the buccal surface or in the heterolateral side of the mandible), make the diagnosis of mandibular osteoradionecrosis more likely [24]. Apart from cortical interruptions, MRI also shows altered bone marrow signal intensities in the involved parts of the mandible [25].

Laryngeal necrosis

Persisting severe edema and radionecrosis of the larynx are uncommon treatment complications, with an incidence of approximately 1%. The occurrence of laryngeal necrosis peaks during the 12 months following treatment, which is more or less contemporaneous with the peak incidence of tumor recurrence. Laryngeal necrosis and tumor recurrence may occur simultaneously. However, cases of laryngeal necrosis occurring more than 10 years after radiation treatment do occur. These late effects after radiation treatment are largely a result of impaired vascular and lymphatic flow, caused by endothelial damage and fibrosis after irradiation. Cartilage itself is resistant to the effect of irradiation; cartilage changes usually occur when the perichondrium is broached by trauma or tumor, exposing the underlying irradiated cartilage to microorganisms in the airway; this may lead to infectious perichondritis, eventually resulting in necrosis and laryngeal collapse.

Patients with laryngeal necrosis often have neck and/or ear pain, some degree of dysphagia and anterior neck swelling.

On imaging studies, a variable degree of laryngeal soft-tissue swelling is seen [26]. These soft-tissue changes surrounding the necrotic cartilage can be very pronounced and may be the only visible abnormality, making the differentiation with recurrent tumor very difficult. In laryngeal necrosis, some fluid may be seen surrounding the cartilages. Cartilaginous abnormalities are often visible, but in some patients they may only become apparent on follow-up CT studies.

Necrosis of the thyroid cartilage may lead to fragmentation and eventually collapse of this cartilage, with or without gas bubbles visible adjacent to it (Fig. 8.6). Patients with arytenoid cartilage necrosis may show anterior dislocation and/or progressive lysis of this cartilage. Also, sloughing of the arytenoid cartilage into the airway may occur [26]. Progressive cricoidal sclerosis may be also seen.

By MRI, laryngeal necrosis may appear as focal swelling of the laryngeal soft tissues, loss of the normal high signal in the medullary space of ossified laryngeal cartilage on T_1-weighted images, and enhancement of the affected cartilage after injection of gadolinium.

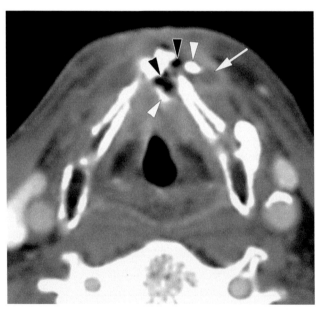

Fig. 8.6. This patient was treated 29 years previously by radiotherapy for a T_1 glottic squamous cell carcinoma. For the previous 6 weeks, the patient has suffered hoarseness, pain and dysphagia. Clinical examination showed a stenotic larynx. Axial contrast-enhanced image shows fragmentation (white arrowheads) of the anterior part of the thyroid cartilage, fluid adjacent to the cartilage (arrow) and small gas bubbles (black arrowheads). These findings are suggestive for laryngeal necrosis. Surgical debridement and reconstruction by placement of a soft tissue flap over the larynx was performed. Symptoms resolved and the patient kept a functional larynx.

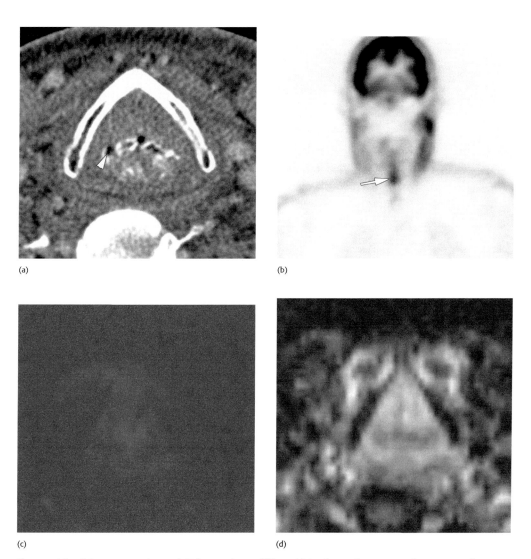

Fig. 8.7. (a) Axial contrast-enhanced CT image shows diffuse thickening and contrast-enhancement of the vocal cords, without focal nodular mass; a small air-bubble can be seen adjacent to the right arytenoid (arrowhead). (b) Coronal FDG PET shows equivocal tracer uptake at the laryngeal level (arrow). (c) No asymmetric hyperintensity is revealed by diffusion-weighted MRI (b1000). (d) The apparent diffusion coefficient map shows diffuse hyperintensity of the soft tissues at the same level. After laryngectomy, histological examination showed necrosis, inflammation and purulent infiltration, without evidence for tumor recurrence.

The use of FDG PET does not seem to be helpful in differentiating laryngeal necrosis from tumor recurrence.

Recently, it was shown that viable tumor in the larynx can be differentiated from necrotic tissue with diffusion-weighted MRI (Fig. 8.7) [13].

Other complications after radiotherapy

Other long-term complications of radiotherapy, occasionally requiring imaging, include soft tissue fibrosis, arteriopathy, delayed central nervous system reaction, radiation myelopathy, cranial nerve palsy and secondary tumors [27].

Conclusions

Post-treatment CT or MRI is of value when a recurrent tumor is suspected, to confirm the presence of such a lesion and to determine its extent. More rarely, imaging may be of use in the differentiation between tumor recurrence and treatment complications.

In patients with a high-risk profile for tumor recurrence after treatment, imaging is of value for surveillance of the patient, as an adjunct to clinical follow-up. The baseline study should be obtained approximately 3 to 4 months after the end of therapy. There is evidence that tumor recurrences can be detected earlier by systematic follow-up imaging, possibly improving patient survival.

REFERENCES

1. S. K. Mukherji, A. A. Mancuso, I. M. Kotzur, *et al.* Radiologic appearance of the irradiated larynx. Part I. Expected changes. *Radiology* **193** (1994), 141–148.
2. P. M. Som, H. D. Curtin, A. A. Mancuso. An imaging-based classification for the cervical nodes designed as an adjunct to recent clinically based nodal classifications. *Arch Otolaryngol Head Neck Surg* **125** (1999), 388–396.
3. R. Hermans, F. A. Pameijer, A. A. Mancuso, J. T. Parsons, W. M. Mendenhall. Laryngeal or hypopharyngeal squamous cell carcinoma: can follow-up CT after definitive radiation therapy be used to detect local failure earlier than clinical examination alone? *Radiology* **214** (2000), 683–687.
4. D. L. Schwartz, J. Barker Jr., K. Chansky, *et al.* Postradiotherapy surveillance practice for head and neck squamous cell carcinoma: too much for too little? *Head Neck* **25** (2003), 990–999.
5. G. B. van den Broek, C. R. Rasch, F. A. Pameijer, *et al.* Response measurement after intraarterial chemoradiation in advanced head and neck carcinoma: magnetic resonance imaging and evaluation under general anesthesia? *Cancer* **106** (2006), 1722–1729.

6. S. K. Mukherji, G. T. Wolf. Evaluation of head and neck squamous cell carcinoma after treatment. *Am J Neuroradiol* **24** (2003), 1743–1746.

7. C. H. Terhaard, V. Bongers, P. P. van Rijk, G. J. Hordijk. F-18-Fluoro-deoxy-glucose positron-emission tomography scanning in detection of local recurrence after radiotherapy for laryngeal/pharyngeal cancer. *Head Neck* **23** (2001), 933–941.

8. Y. Kitagawa, S. Nishizawa, K. Sano, *et al.* Prospective comparison of 18F-FDG PET with conventional imaging modalities (MRI, CT, and ^{67}Ga scintigraphy) in assessment of combined intraarterial chemotherapy and radiotherapy for head and neck carcinoma. *J Nucl Med* **44** (2003), 198–206.

9. K. Kubota, J. Yokoyama, K. Yamaguchi, *et al.* FDG-PET delayed imaging for the detection of head and neck cancer recurrence after radio-chemotherapy: comparison with MRI/CT. *Eur J Nucl Med Mol Imaging* **31** (2004), 590–595.

10. R. S. Andrade, D. E. Heron, B. Degirmenci, *et al.* Posttreatment assessment of response using FDG-PET/CT for patients treated with definitive radiation therapy for head and neck cancers. *Int J Radiat Oncol Biol Phys* **65** (2006), 1315–1322.

11. B. F. Branstetter, T. M. Blodgett, L. A. Zimmer, *et al.* Head and neck malignancy: is PET/CT more accurate than PET or CT alone? *Radiology* **235** (2005), 580–586.

12. H. C. Thoeny, F. De Keyzer, F. Chen, *et al.* Diffusion-weighted MR imaging in monitoring the effect of a vascular targeting agent on rhabdomyosarcoma in rats. *Radiology* **234** (2005), 756–764.

13. V. Vandecaveye, F. de Keyzer, V. Vander Poorten, *et al.* Evaluation of the larynx for tumor recurrence by diffusion-weighted MRI after radiotherapy: initial experience in four cases. *Br J Radiol* **79** (2006), 681–687.

14. V. Vandecaveye, F. de Keyzer, S. Nuyts, *et al.* Detection of head and neck squamous cell carcinoma with diffusion weighted MRI after (chemo)radiotherapy: correlation between radiologic and histopathologic findings. *Int J Radiat Oncol Biol Phys* **67** (2007), 960–971.

15. P. K. Pellitteri, A. Ferlito, A. Rinaldo, *et al.* Planned neck dissection following chemoradiotherapy for advanced head and neck cancer: is it necessary for all? *Head Neck* **28** (2006), 166–175.

16. S. L. Liauw, A. A. Mancuso, R. J. Amdur, *et al.* Postradiotherapy neck dissection for lymph node-positive head and neck cancer: the use of computed tomography to manage the neck. *J Clin Oncol* **24** (2006), 1421–1427.

17. J. W. Rogers, K. M. Greven, W. F. McGuirt, *et al.* Can post-RT neck dissection be omitted for patients with head-and-neck cancer who have a negative PET scan after definitive radiation therapy? *Int J Radiat Oncol Biol Phys* **58** (2004), 694–697.

18. C. Castaigne, K. Muylle, P. Flamen. Positron emission tomography in head and neck cancer. In *Head and Neck Cancer Imaging*, ed. R. Hermans (Berlin: Springer, 2006), pp. 329–343.

19. M. Yao, M. M. Graham, H. T. Hoffman, *et al.* The role of post-radiation therapy FDG PET in prediction of necessity for post-radiation therapy neck dissection in locally advanced head-and-neck squamous cell carcinoma. *Int J Radiat Oncol Biol Phys* **59** (2004), 1001–1010.

20. S. V. Porceddu, E. Jarmolowski, R. J. Hicks, *et al.* Utility of positron emission tomography for the detection of disease in residual neck nodes after (chemo)radiotherapy in head and neck cancer. *Head Neck* **27** (2005), 175–181.

21. A. V. de Visscher, J. J. Manni. Routine long-term follow-up in patients treated with curative intent for squamous cell carcinoma of the larynx, pharynx, and oral cavity. Does it make sense? *Arch Otolaryngol Head Neck Surg* **120** (1994), 934–939.

22. T. R. Cooney, M. G. Poulsen. Is routine follow-up useful after combined-modality therapy for advanced head and neck cancer? *Arch Otolaryngol Head Neck Surg* **125** (1999), 379–382.

23. R. E. Marx. Osteoradionecrosis: a new concept of its pathophysiology. *J Oral Maxillofac Surg* **41** (1983), 283–288.

24. R. Hermans. Imaging of mandibular osteoradionecrosis. *Neuroimaging Clin North Am* **13** (2003), 597–604.

25. J. Chong, L. K. Hinckley, L. E. Ginsberg. Masticator space abnormalities associated with mandibular osteoradionecrosis: MR and CT findings in five patients. *Am J Neuroradiol* **21** (2000), 175–178.

26. R. Hermans, F. A. Pameijer, A. A. Mancuso, J. T. Parsons, W. M. Mendenhall. CT findings in chondroradionecrosis of the larynx. *Am J Neuroradiol* **19** (1998), 711–718.

27. M. Becker, G. Schroth, P. Zbaren, *et al.* Long-term changes induced by high-dose irradiation of the head and neck region: imaging findings. *Radiographics* **17** (1997), 5–26.

Index